Overcoming Low Self-esteem
with Mindfulness

Deborah Ward is a writer and editor whose passion for personal growth and psychology has led to the publication of numerous feature articles for a variety of print and online magazines. With a desire to nurture the personal development, self-esteem and potential of others, she also writes a regular blog called Sense and Sensitivity for *Psychology Today* magazine, on the subject of coping with high sensitivity. Deborah's creative interests also include writing fiction. She has published numerous short stories and is currently also working on a novel. Through her writing, Deborah strives to provide the clarity and compassion both to inspire others to be their true selves and to shed light on issues that are so often hidden in darkness. She is the author of *Overcoming Fear with Mindfulness*, also published by Sheldon Press (2013).

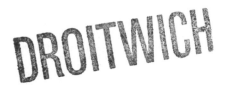

Overcoming Common Problems Series

Selected titles

A full list of titles is available from Sheldon Press,
36 Causton Street, London SW1P 4ST and on our website at
www.sheldonpress.co.uk

Overcoming Common Problems Series

Overcoming Common Problems Series

Living with Tinnitus and Hyperacusis
Dr Laurence McKenna, Dr David Baguley
and Dr Don McFerran

Losing a Parent
Fiona Marshall

**Making Sense of Trauma: How to tell
your story**
Dr Nigel C. Hunt and Dr Sue McHale

Menopause in Perspective
Philippa Pigache

Motor Neurone Disease: A family affair
Dr David Oliver

The Multiple Sclerosis Diet Book
Tessa Buckley

Natural Treatments for Arthritis
Christine Craggs-Hinton

Overcome Your Fear of Flying
Professor Robert Bor, Dr Carina Eriksen
and Margaret Oakes

Overcoming Anorexia
Professor J. Hubert Lacey, Christine Craggs-Hinton
and Kate Robinson

Overcoming Emotional Abuse
Susan Elliot-Wright

Overcoming Fear: With mindfulness
Deborah Ward

**Overcoming Gambling: A guide for problem
and compulsive gamblers**
Philip Mawer

Overcoming Hurt
Dr Windy Dryden

Overcoming Jealousy
Dr Windy Dryden

Overcoming Loneliness
Alice Muir

**Overcoming Panic and Related Anxiety
Disorders**
Margaret Hawkins

Overcoming Procrastination
Dr Windy Dryden

Overcoming Shyness and Social Anxiety
Dr Ruth Searle

Overcoming Stress
Professor Robert Bor, Dr Carina Eriksen
and Dr Sara Chaudry

Overcoming Worry and Anxiety
Dr Jerry Kennard

**The Pain Management Handbook:
Your personal guide**
Neville Shone

The Panic Workbook
Dr Carina Eriksen, Professor Robert Bor
and Margaret Oakes

**Physical Intelligence: How to take charge of
your weight**
Dr Tom Smith

Reducing Your Risk of Dementia
Dr Tom Smith

**Self-discipline: How to get it and how to
keep it**
Dr Windy Dryden

The Self-Esteem Journal
Alison Waines

Sinusitis: Steps to healing
Dr Paul Carson

Stammering: Advice for all ages
Renée Byrne and Louise Wright

Stress-related Illness
Dr Tim Cantopher

The Stroke Survival Guide
Mark Greener

Ten Steps to Positive Living
Dr Windy Dryden

**Therapy for Beginners: How to get the best
out of counselling**
Professor Robert Bor, Sheila Gill and Anne Stokes

Think Your Way to Happiness
Dr Windy Dryden and Jack Gordon

**Tranquillizers and Antidepressants: When to
take them, how to stop**
Professor Malcolm Lader

**Transforming Eight Deadly Emotions
into Healthy Ones**
Dr Windy Dryden

The Traveller's Good Health Guide
Dr Ted Lankester

Treating Arthritis Diet Book
Margaret Hills

Treating Arthritis: The drug-free way
Margaret Hills and Christine Horner

Treating Arthritis: More ways to a drug-free life
Margaret Hills

Treating Arthritis: The supplements guide
Julia Davies

Understanding Obsessions and Compulsions
Dr Frank Tallis

Understanding Traumatic Stress
Dr Nigel Hunt and Dr Sue McHale

**Understanding Yourself and Others:
Practical ideas from the world of coaching**
Bob Thomson

When Someone You Love Has Dementia
Susan Elliot-Wright

**When Someone You Love Has Depression:
A handbook for family and friends**
Barbara Baker

Overcoming Common Problems

Overcoming Low Self-esteem with Mindfulness

DEBORAH WARD

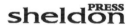

First published in Great Britain in 2015

Sheldon Press
36 Causton Street
London SW1P 4ST
www.sheldonpress.co.uk

British Library Cataloguing-in-Publication Data
A catalogue record for this book is available from the British Library

ISBN 978–1–84709–345–5
eBook ISBN 978–1–84709–346–2

Typeset by Fakenham Prepress Solutions, Fakenham, Norfolk NR21 8NN
First printed in Great Britain by Ashford Colour Press
Subsequently digitally printed in Great Britain

eBook by Fakenham Prepress Solutions, Fakenham, Norfolk NR21 8NN

Produced on paper from sustainable forests

Contents

Introduction

Susan was a happily married woman who worked for a large accounting firm. She also did volunteer work and enjoyed helping her neighbours and being part of the community. When anyone needed help, they knew they could always come to Susan. Even Susan's friends, her boss and her husband Tom felt that way. She felt good when people said they needed her help and she didn't like to disappoint anyone.

One day she'd agreed to help with the church fundraiser by baking a cake, but at the event she felt that hers wasn't very good. Instead of enjoying the fundraiser Susan hovered in a corner, willing herself to disappear, wishing she could run away and silently chastising herself for doing such a terrible job.

Her husband Tom often worked late hours but enjoyed his job and felt motivated to work hard because he wanted to support his family. He could never quite believe Susan had agreed to marry him – she was so beautiful, and deep down he knew she was too good for him. Susan liked to have things a certain way at home and Tom always agreed with her preferences and requests because he thought he owed her. He wanted to make her happy. If he wasn't proving himself to be the best husband and father, the best provider, the best at everything, he just knew she'd leave him. Every day he struggled to prove to her he was good enough but somehow, no matter how hard he worked, he never felt he was.

Perhaps no other self-help topic has spawned so much advice and so many conflicting theories as self-esteem. Healthy self-esteem gives us the ability to make positive choices regarding our career and our relationships, and gives us the assertiveness and confidence to work towards our goals. Overly high self-esteem is not healthy, however, as it can lead to a sense of entitlement, as well as bullying and narcissistic behaviour. A lack of self-esteem can lead to a life of putting up with abusive situations or relationships, depression and lack of fulfilment.

Our personalities, according to Sigmund Freud, emerge out of our struggles to meet our needs in a world that often frustrates these efforts. Our self-esteem develops, grows and changes according to our success or failure in that struggle and the often self-defeating ways we attempt to cope. With the tools of mindfulness, however, we can improve our self-esteem while finding new and healthier ways to get our needs met.

By working on self-esteem with mindfulness, which has been defined by Jon Kabat-Zinn as paying attention in a particular way, this book offers readers the choice to break out of the unconscious thought and behaviour patterns that create unsatisfactory lives, and to achieve real freedom, fulfilment and happiness.

What is low self-esteem?

According to Marilyn Sorensen, the director of the Self-Esteem Institute in Portland, Oregon, low self-esteem is a thinking disorder in which individuals see themselves as inadequate, unacceptable, unworthy, unlovable, and/or incompetent. These beliefs create thoughts that tend to be negative, self-critical, self-blaming and full of self-doubt. And these thoughts consequently affect our behaviour, leading to destructive patterns of avoidance, denial, criticism and defensiveness that lower our self-esteem even further.

Low self-esteem is a basic tendency to place one's value in the hands of others, rather than trusting and believing in our own evaluation of ourselves. When your self-esteem depends on other people's view of you, it only makes it more fragile. Thoughts follow that are also irrational and distorted, causing you to have difficulty knowing whom to trust and when to trust, inciting fear and anxiety in new situations or assuming other people think as negatively of you as you do.

Low self-esteem affects every aspect of our lives, from our career choices to our relationships with friends, family and loved ones. All too often we don't even realize that our own feelings of low self-worth are affecting us because they're largely subconscious, quietly influencing the choices we make and creating a life that leaves us feeling unaccepted, unworthy and unloved. When we have low self-esteem it can be very easy to think our lives are unfulfilling or unhappy because we don't deserve the good fortune, happiness and success of others. But it's our negative beliefs and self-critical thinking that lead us to such negative views.

Learning to recognize and identify the symptoms of low self-esteem in yourself is the first step. Some of these symptoms can include:

- depression
- discouragement
- fear and anxiety
- emotional shutdown
- panic attacks
- social anxiety
- eating disorders
- lack of assertiveness
- passive-aggression
- people-pleasing
- controlling behaviour.

How does low self-esteem affect your life?

When we feel we're not good enough or are flawed or unlovable, we'll act in ways that not only *reflect* these beliefs but *reinforce* them. We might:

- avoid opportunities for advancement at work;
- settle for less than we deserve;
- fail to assert our needs or desires;
- apologize constantly and try to please everyone;
- choose people who support our negative view of ourselves;
- find it difficult to leave relationships even when we're unhappy;
- control others to try to prevent them from controlling us;
- find it difficult to relax and enjoy ourselves, feeling we don't deserve it or we have to work harder to prove ourselves to others;
- neglect ourselves by overworking, overeating, spending too much money, drinking too much or taking drugs.

This kind of behaviour leads us to believe that we're the unworthy people we believed ourselves to be, creating feelings of sadness, guilt, shame, frustration or anger and lowering our self-esteem. Research has found that people with genuine low self-esteem tend to treat themselves badly, not other people, at least not intentionally. But when you don't see yourself as someone deserving of love, respect and support, other people won't either, and you can quickly find yourself in unhealthy relationships.

According to Marilyn Sorensen, people with low self-esteem often feel fearful and anxious. For some this fear can escalate into panic attacks, so that they withdraw and isolate themselves socially as they struggle to cope with feeling embarrassed, depressed or despairing. Usually they're too fearful to ask for help, believing doing so would be an admission of failure.

What causes low self-esteem?

Our poor self-image and feelings of low self-worth come from our early experiences – we're not born with low self-esteem. If as children we're the object of anger, abandonment, neglect, abuse or continual criticism, we'll accept those perceptions of ourselves as true. Children believe what they're taught, so if parents mistreat them, they'll believe they deserve it. If parents don't show love or affection, children will believe they're unlovable. This negative view of ourselves stays with us and affects every aspect of our lives, as we continue to see ourselves based on the rejecting, critical behaviour of others rather than the truth of who we are.

As we grow up, even someone with healthy self-esteem can feel suddenly shattered when faced with life's challenges, including bullying or social rejection at school. As adults our self-esteem can waver under the influence of job loss, divorce, death of a loved one, financial worries, physical or mental health problems or any traumatic situations.

Negative beliefs about ourselves are difficult to change because our childhood experiences define what is 'normal' for each of us. For people whose upbringing included criticism, contempt, anger or other destructive environments, healthy behaviour may be something they neither recognize nor have any idea how to achieve.

What is healthy self-esteem?

Building healthy self-esteem comes from learning to value ourselves and not depending on other people's opinions of us. This dependence on approval causes us to keep trying to get love and acceptance from people who are unlikely to give it, thus perpetuating our negative beliefs about ourselves.

People with healthy self-esteem don't worry about what others may be thinking of them – they assume others think as well of them as they think of themselves. They speak their minds and express themselves openly without fear of judgement, rejection or ridicule.

According to Sorensen, people with healthy self-esteem can admit their mistakes or their inabilities and ask for help without feeling embarrassed or inadequate. They believe they can meet challenges that arise and cope with life. Likewise they don't fear they'll lose what they have and they believe they deserve it, whether it's career success, relationships or happiness.

Here are some signs of someone with healthy self-esteem. He or she:

- sets attainable goals;
- doesn't procrastinate or become a perfectionist;
- accepts his or her weaknesses;
- is highly motivated and able to overcome obstacles;
- bounces back after a setback;
- asserts himself or herself and expresses his or her own ideas, feelings and opinions;
- is open to and learns from constructive criticism without feeling attacked;
- engages with others socially;
- learns from past mistakes;
- is able to take risks;
- knows whom to trust.

To develop your self-esteem you need to let go of childlike ways of coping, which means no longer depending on other people's approval. Over time you learn to become the parent to yourself, to love yourself the way you've always needed to be loved and to come to believe in your own assessment of yourself rather than needing to seek the appraisal of others.

Overcoming low self-esteem requires an awareness of your negative thoughts, feelings and behaviour and then choosing how to respond to them rather than simply reacting to them out of fear.

Once you develop awareness, you can work on bringing acceptance to your experience, accepting the thoughts as just thoughts, accepting the emotions they trigger, and gradually accepting yourself as you are.

How mindfulness can help

When you are mindful you're able to look at things, situations and people objectively, without judgement and without the negative influence of the past. When you are mindful you see only the present moment, free from the fears of the past and the anxieties about the future, and realize you have a choice. You have the choice to stay or to go, to work harder or work differently, to move forward or to change direction. What's important is to choose what's right for you, based on your values, needs and goals, instead of reacting based on what you believe others will think of you.

Non-judgemental awareness

Mindfulness allows you to develop a gentle awareness of your thoughts, feelings and beliefs and to see them as objects, rather than interpreting them as illustrations of who you are. Mindfulness can help you to wake up from the bad dream of negative thinking and see where your own thoughts, beliefs and reactions have led to poor choices. It allows you to clear out the clutter in your mind that's muddied your thinking and to see the truth of who you are and what is happening, so you can make healthy choices for yourself.

A recent study in the journal *Perspectives on Psychological Science* showed that mindfulness can help us to know ourselves better. Researchers suggested that non-judgemental observation of our thoughts, feelings and behaviour can reduce our tendency to react emotionally, such as with feelings of inadequacy, shame or guilt, which limits our ability to see the truth about ourselves. The study also showed that mindfulness can help develop our bodily awareness, so we can recognize our own nonverbal behaviour, such as fidgeting or nail biting or other signs of anxiety.

Non-attachment

Many of us struggle to overcome low self-esteem because we've spent our lives believing the negative thoughts we have about ourselves. We may have tried to deal with these by repeating positive statements, such as 'I'm a loveable person'. But researchers have found that people with low self-esteem actually feel worse after repeating positive statements about themselves. These statements, whether spoken to yourself or by someone else, contradict the beliefs low self-esteem people have about themselves – the participants in the research could not accept them. The positive statements did not help because they didn't believe they were true.

In her research on low self-esteem, Melanie Fennell asserts that mindfulness meditation leads to enhanced 'metacognitive awareness'; that is, an ability to experience thoughts as transient mental events rather than as aspects of the self or reflections of truth. This doesn't mean we look at our thoughts or feelings coldly or impassively, but with kindness and acceptance and as separate from ourselves, and free from self-criticism – the way we might look at a tree, a horse or a cloud.

When we connect ourselves to our thoughts and feelings we end up comparing ourselves to others and consequently feel jealousy, envy, embarrassment or anger. By offering ourselves a compassionate, mindful perspective on our negative thoughts and beliefs and letting them go, we can come to see them as separate from ourselves and accept ourselves as we are.

Compassion

Compassion is an essential element of mindfulness. Recent research by Juliana Breines and Serena Chen has shown that treating yourself with compassion after making a mistake increases your motivation to develop self-improvement. The study showed that taking an accepting approach to personal failure can help people to become more motivated to improve themselves.

Mindful meditation can train your brain to develop your motivational skills, including attention, focus, stress management, impulse control and self-awareness. Studies show that changes in the brain have been observed after only eight weeks of daily meditation.

Another study from researchers at Northeastern and Harvard Universities suggested that meditation can also make us more compassionate towards others. The findings showed that volunteers who underwent eight-week training in two types of meditation reacted more compassionately than those who hadn't meditated.

Perhaps most importantly, developing compassion for yourself allows you to let go of your own negative beliefs and to see yourself as someone who deserves to be loved, accepted and appreciated. When you're compassionate you can offer that love and acceptance to yourself.

Living in the moment

Mindfulness techniques can help you stay focused in the present moment. Over time these techniques build your ability to stay mindful, in the same way regular exercise builds muscle and endurance levels. These techniques include meditation, deep breathing, mindful walking and yoga. These practices don't have to be complicated – they simply involve focusing on the moment through an awareness of your body and your breathing, while quieting your mind and letting go of any distracting thoughts.

Mindfulness techniques such as deep breathing and meditation also lower stress, causing you not only to feel calmer but decreasing levels of the stress hormone cortisol. When you're calm you can consciously choose how to respond to anxiety-triggering situations rather than immediately taking action you may later regret. In this way you not only feel more relaxed, you're taking control of your behaviour and choosing the life you want – a process that builds self-esteem through one positive experience after another. According to the clinical psychologist Joseph Burgo, author of *Why Do I Do That?*, it's only by making a different choice, over and over, that you'll begin to develop new habits.

How to read this book

Each chapter in this book will examine a different symptom and consequence of low self-esteem as well as a corresponding characteristic of mindfulness. While the symptoms of low self-esteem presented here are not exhaustive, many of these conditions are common and they often interact. Some people will exhibit all of these symptoms and others only one or two. But each chapter will show you how to turn those negative behaviours, beliefs and feelings into something positive that builds your self-esteem using mindfulness techniques, allowing you to see how change occurs not only with awareness, but with choice.

As you learn about each characteristic of mindfulness and how you can use it to develop your own self-esteem, you'll see how they work together to create a new way of looking at the world and at yourself. With compassion, acceptance and a non-judgemental way of focusing on the present moment, you'll develop an awareness of what is really happening in your life, along with a loving, compassionate acceptance of who you are. With mindful practice you'll be free of the stranglehold of your past experiences and able to make your own choices regarding your work, your love, your life and your beliefs about yourself. When you're mindful you'll be offering yourself the love and acceptance you always wanted and building your self-esteem from one moment to the next.

1

Self-loathing or self-compassion

Treat yourself with love and compassion and gentleness, the way you would any child . . . When you do, you'll feel loved and be loved.

Tom was trying for a promotion at work. He knew that if he could get it, it would mean more money and then he could finish the renovations on the house and maybe even buy that holiday home in Spain Susan had been talking about. He'd worked hard and felt he deserved a promotion, but as he stood outside the meeting room on Monday morning waiting to give his presentation, his mind was racing with negative thoughts.

'I'm going to screw this up,' he thought, 'I'm terrible at speaking in front of other people. I don't know why I thought I could do it.'

As he shuffled through his notes, he heard his father's voice: 'What are you doing? You'll never get it right. Why do you even bother?'

As the meeting room door opened, Tom felt his hands shake and his forehead begin to sweat. Images of his father's and his wife's disappointed faces flashed across his mind, and as he smiled and walked into the room, all he could feel was an overwhelming sense of inadequacy and self-hatred that blurred his thinking.

What is self-loathing?

The lack of love for yourself, or self-loathing, is at the root of low self-esteem. We hate ourselves because we believe we're inadequate and unlovable. We compare ourselves to others and find ourselves lacking. We're unable to accept compliments. We can't forgive ourselves for the smallest of mistakes because they're evidence of our incompetence. Consequently we're plagued by feelings of frustration and anger and deep-rooted feelings of shame about who we are.

Why do we hate ourselves?

Self-loathing is not the result of your inadequacy, failure, incompetence or unlovableness. It's the result of thinking of yourself that way. We think that way because those thoughts and ideas and beliefs were planted in our minds when we were growing up. For any number of reasons, we felt unworthy, unacceptable or unloved because of the way we were treated or spoken to. When rejection comes from a parent, we believe it as truth.

Sometimes a harsh or chaotic environment can create feelings of anxiety and fear in children as a way of coping. When home life is unpredictable, constantly changing or the caregivers are unreliable, such as when food, shelter or money is inconsistent or the family moves a lot, children can easily blame themselves and develop self-hatred.

As we grow up it becomes very difficult to challenge those beliefs, partly because we're often completely unaware of them. They become such a deep-rooted part of our lives that when others suggest we're in fact good enough, we can feel uncomfortable and resistant to the very idea. It's also difficult to change these beliefs because we ourselves believe they're true. Consequently we live our lives looking for evidence to support this negative belief and discounting any evidence to the contrary.

In her research Kristin Neff, an expert in human development and self-compassion, found that the main reason people aren't more compassionate towards themselves is that they feel they need to be tough on themselves to get ahead. They believe compassion would only make them self-indulgent. According to Neff, many people believe self-criticism is the right thing to do because our culture encourages being hard on yourself and getting ahead through self-discipline and deprivation, whether you're trying to climb the corporate ladder, get a second date or lose 20 pounds. However, studies have shown that self-criticism can lower self-esteem and increase anxiety and depression. In addition, self-criticism assumes you're 'bad' and increases your fear of failure.

Another reason why we find it difficult to have compassion for ourselves, according to the psychologists Susan Orsillo and Lizabeth Roemer, is that we believe our thoughts have power. When thoughts emerge we focus on them and try to find solutions to their problems, in the belief that if we don't solve them they won't go away. But this strategy usually results only in worry, partly because many problems are out of our control and partly because our thoughts aren't always based on truth but on our negative beliefs.

How does self-loathing affect us?

If we believe we're unworthy of love we tend to push away love when it comes to us – it feels so unfamiliar and so untrue that our subconscious mind believes it must be dangerous. Sometimes we simply avoid relationships or getting close to others to keep them from seeing the 'truth' about how unworthy we really are. Despite all our efforts to conceal the way we really feel about ourselves, deep down we feel we're not good enough for others, that we don't really deserve to be loved unconditionally, we don't deserve respect, and so we abandon loving relationships and often pursue unhealthy relationships with people who treat us the way we believe we deserve. At its most extreme, people who hate themselves can succumb to substance abuse, suicide and other self-destructive behaviours, as well as violence towards others.

Self-loathers think they know themselves better than anyone else does, says the philosopher Mark D. White, which is why they believe they can see their own negative qualities while other people can't. They believe others simply can't see the real person with all his or her flaws. This is why trying to boost someone's self-esteem with praise doesn't work – the self-loathing person doesn't believe it and thinks the other person just doesn't see the truth.

A person with low self-esteem is often riddled with shame. When you feel you're not good enough you blame yourself for your inadequacies and feel ashamed of who you are. As a consequence, those who do not love themselves will tend to put themselves down, sometimes only to prevent others from doing so. According to the clinical psychologist Joseph Burgo, such people are actually trying to gain control over an experience they would find devastating.

The mindful way – self-compassion

The Dalai Lama defines compassion as a non-judgemental openness to the suffering of oneself and others with a strong desire to alleviate suffering in all living things. Mindfulness encourages us to be aware of ourselves, our thoughts, our feelings and our surroundings, and to look at them in a gentle, loving, caring way, without judgement. This is compassion. And we can be more compassionate to others when we first show that compassion to ourselves.

Studies show that the more compassionate we are towards ourselves, the more compassion we show to others. One study revealed that when therapists rated how compassionate or critical they were with themselves, their ratings matched their compassion towards their patients.

Showing compassion towards yourself is a fundamental part of mindfulness in which you accept that you deserve love as much as anyone else. It's not about being selfish or self-pitying. It's providing yourself with the love, safety and acceptance you need to grow and flourish without fear.

When you're struggling to feel loved you're trying to *get* love from others and consequently you have nothing to *give*. When you love yourself you no longer feel the need to fight for what you want, to get defensive, push others away or compare yourself with other people. You simply accept yourself as you are in a loving, non-judgemental way. You can then begin to share the love and acceptance you feel for yourself with others because you have everything you need.

> A week after his presentation at work, Tom was sitting outside his boss's office, waiting for a meeting to discuss his possible promotion. His boss always started meetings late – on purpose, Tom thought, to make him feel anxious. He rubbed his sweating hands on his knees. 'I'm not going to get the promotion,' he thought. 'I've screwed it up – I knew I would.' Then he took a deep breath and exhaled slowly. 'Okay,' he thought, 'it's normal to be nervous about a promotion. Everyone gets nervous. Have I screwed it up? Well, I've worked hard and done my best so that's all I can do. I'm proud of myself for the job I've done. And I know Susan is proud of me too. Whatever happens, I'll be okay.'

In her article 'Self-Compassion: An Alternative Conceptualization of a Healthy Attitude Toward Oneself', the researcher Kristin Neff has outlined three main aspects of self-compassion:

1 *Self-kindness* – extending kindness and understanding to oneself rather than harsh judgement and self-criticism;

2   *Common humanity* – seeing one's experiences as part of the larger human experience rather than as separating and isolating;
3   *Mindfulness* – holding one's painful thoughts and feelings in balanced awareness rather than over-identifying with them.

It can be very difficult for self-loathing people to begin to feel self-compassion, however, because they simply don't believe they deserve it. Many people with low self-esteem live in a constant state of fear, either fear of a threatening external world of people who could criticize, reject, abandon or abuse them, or because of their own internal fears and self-criticisms.

A recent study by Ibrahim Senay, Dolores Albarracín and Kenji Noguchi in the journal *Psychological Science* has revealed that positive affirmations or telling yourself positive statements, such as 'I'm good', 'I'm worthy', 'I'm great at my job', are intended to boost your self-confidence but fail to boost self-esteem. The study showed that affirmations tend to apply pressure to ourselves and create a fear of failure that shuts down our ability to look at the situation and ourselves objectively and compassionately. If you don't believe you're good or worthy, telling yourself you are won't be motivating because you think it's untrue. It becomes too easy simply to ignore such positive statements when they don't fit with your understanding of who you believe yourself to be.

When people asked themselves questions instead of telling themselves statements, however, the researchers found a significant difference. Questions demand answers and consequently stimulate our minds to come up with possibilities, which may be numerous. If there are possibilities there is potential for change. If you're nervous about a presentation at work, for example, you may find yourself thinking, 'I'm going to mess this up. I'm terrible at presentations.' But if you instead ask the question, 'Am I terrible at presentations?' you'll probably come up with examples of how anxious you feel as well as examples of your skills and abilities that have worked well.

According to the researchers, this strategy works because it acknowledges your negative thoughts and feelings and allows you to accept yourself with your flaws rather than fighting them. In addition, once you start asking questions, you're no longer accepting a single statement as truth, such as 'I'm bad', but allowing yourself to see your difficult thoughts and feelings as temporary objects rather than aspects of yourself. Once you start asking more questions, such as 'What did I do right in the last presentation?', 'How can I learn from my evaluation?' and 'What if I organized my notes differently next time?' you'll be able to accept your nervousness and anxiety with compassion while moving forward without fear.

Feeling safe, cared for and loved can feel threatening. But studies have shown that self-compassion can help people overcome feelings of shame and self-criticism. The key is to recognize that these negative thoughts and feelings were planted by people in your past. Someone told you or made you believe you weren't good enough. What you need to recognize now is that they were wrong. They expressed an opinion, not the truth. As a child you believe what adults tell you; as an adult you can decide for yourself. You're good enough; you deserve compassion; and you deserve love.

Self-kindness

If you never got the love and acceptance you needed in the past, you'll be looking for it in your relationships with other people. But you can't get that true love if you don't believe you deserve it, so you push it away when it's offered, or stay with people who don't love you. But you can give that love to yourself.

What does it mean to love yourself? Instead of judging yourself harshly with blame and self-criticism, such as telling yourself you're inadequate or a failure, offer yourself love and kindness. Become the loving adult to the child within you. Be your own parent and take care of yourself. Treat yourself with love and compassion and gentleness, the way you would any child. In his book *Compassion and Self-Hate*, the psychiatrist Theodore I. Rubin advises readers to tell themselves, 'I treat myself as I treat a child I love.' Tell yourself you're all right, things will be all right, and that you're loved. When you do, you'll feel loved and be loved.

According to the clinical psychologist and mindfulness expert Shauna Shapiro, self-kindness also means you allow yourself to experience your feelings and to respond to them with kindness. So even if you're feeling angry, hurt, sad or frustrated, you can be aware of those feelings and simply accept them as natural human emotions without criticizing or judging yourself for having them.

Blaming yourself or getting angry at yourself for feeling what you feel, only results in stress, frustration and lowered self-esteem.

Common humanity

When things don't go your way you can easily feel a sense of isolation, as if you're the only person who's suffering, explains Kristin Neff. Recognizing that everyone suffers and everyone makes mistakes, however, can allow us to see that we don't need to be hard on ourselves and criticize ourselves for our faults. Instead we can offer the same compassion to ourselves we offer to others when they make mistakes or fail or suffer. Everyone has flaws and that's what makes us all part of the common human experience.

Recognizing our common humanity also means we recognize that our thoughts, feelings and behaviour are all affected by our personal history, environment, culture and genes as well as the behaviour of other people in what the Buddhist monk Thich Nhat Hanh calls 'interbeing'. Because we all affect each other and respond in individual ways to the many influences upon us, we can be compassionate and non-judgemental about our own part in this intricate human interconnection.

Once we accept that there are aspects of life we can't control, we can accept that sometimes we'll have struggles and challenges but we're still acceptable, valuable and essential members of society, just the way we are.

Mindfulness

Changing the beliefs you've held for a lifetime can be difficult. Those beliefs are what drive your behaviour, including the way you behave in relationships, react to various situations and the way you treat yourself. If compassion for yourself is a new experience, it will take practice. Just like learning to play the piano, it's something that requires a conscious choice every day for it to become a habit. But with practice you'll become better at it and find it easier until it becomes a part of who you are.

One of the ways to practise self-compassion is through mindfulness meditation. According to the self-esteem expert Melanie Fennell, mindfulness meditation leads to an enhanced ability to accept that thoughts and beliefs are transient mental events rather than aspects of the self or reflections of truth. No matter what that emotion may be or how intense it may feel, mindfulness meditation can help us recognize that it's not who we are and that it's temporary.

In this way mindfulness can help us become aware of the negative thoughts and beliefs we have about ourselves and recognize that they're separate from who we are. It also allows us to move away from automatic pilot behaviour and instead become able to choose consciously the way we would like to respond to the thoughts that appear in our minds. As Fennell writes, 'The familiar negative view is only one possibility and may be neither the truest nor the most adaptive.'

Loving-kindness meditation with self-compassion

Christopher Germer, a clinical psychologist and author of *The Mindful Path to Self-Compassion*, offers several mindfulness meditations; the one in the panel overleaf is a traditional loving-kindness meditation that focuses on self-compassion.

Learning to be compassionate towards your own responses means you accept that your thoughts and feelings are natural and part of the common human experience rather than criticizing yourself for having them. In their book *The Mindful Way Through Anxiety*, the psychologists Susan Orsillo and Lizabeth Roemer explain that when we continually practise self-compassion as a daily habit, we can break the cycle of reactivity and self-criticism that often creates anxiety and lowers self-esteem.

1 Find a comfortable position, sitting or lying down. Let your
   eyes close, fully or partially. Take a few deep breaths to settle
   into your body and into the present moment. You might like to
   put your hand over your heart, or wherever it's comforting and
   soothing, as a reminder to bring not only awareness, but *loving*
   awareness, to your experience and to yourself.
2 Locate your breathing where you can feel it most easily. Feel
   your breath move through your body, and when your attention
   wanders, feel the gentle movement of your breath once again.
   Let your body breathe you.
3 After a few minutes, start to notice any physical sensations of
   stress that you may be holding in your body, perhaps in your
   neck, jaw, belly or forehead.
4 Notice if you're holding some difficult emotions, such as worry
   about the future or uneasiness about the past. Understand that
   every human body bears stress and worry throughout the day.
5 See if you can move towards the stress in your body as you
   might incline towards a child or a beloved pet, with curiosity
   and tenderness.
6 Now incline towards *yourself*, offering yourself goodwill simply
   because of the stress you're holding in your body right now, as
   everyone holds stress in their bodies. Offering words of kindness
   and compassion to yourself, slowly and affectionately. For
   example:

> May I be safe
> May I be peaceful
> May I be kind to myself
> May I accept myself as I am

7 Whenever you notice that your mind has wandered, return to
   the sensations in your body and to the loving-kindness phrases.
8 If you're ever swept up in emotion, you can always return to
   your breathing. Then, when you're comfortable again, return to
   the phrases.
9 Finally, take a few breaths and just rest quietly in your own body,
   knowing that you can return to the phrases any time you wish.
10 Gently open your eyes.

2

Unhealthy relationships or living in the moment

When you're focused on the moment you can choose your actions consciously and wisely and in a state of calm, rational love, instead of unconscious, reactive fear.

Whenever Susan got into an argument with Tom she felt so hurt and upset she had to leave the room. She'd go to their bedroom and cry, overwhelmed by Tom's criticism of her and her feelings of rejection. She hoped Tom would come in and comfort her, but when he didn't, she felt abandoned. She was sure Tom was arguing with her because he didn't approve of the way she cooked dinner and questioned his whereabouts, and now she had proof he didn't really care about her feelings at all, just as she'd suspected. It was the same way her mother had acted when she was young – nothing was ever good enough for her. Drying her tears, Susan told herself she just had to try harder to win Tom's love.

Our struggles with low self-esteem often make themselves most clearly known in our closest relationships. While we can hide our fears and self-doubts from ourselves, we can't hide them from other people because our reactions and responses to others reveal the way we feel about ourselves. The closer we are to someone, the more we risk getting hurt, so intimate relationships tend to amplify each person's insecurities and personal issues. Unfortunately, people with low self-esteem tend to be attracted to people with similar levels of self-esteem. The result is often a power struggle that creates hurt feelings, misunderstandings, poor communication and sometimes the failure of the relationship that would bring us the love we so desperately want.

What is an unhealthy relationship?

Disagreements and arguments happen in every relationship, but at some stage these can become unhealthy. But how do you know what is healthy and what is not? According to the clinical psychologist Seth Meyers, good relationships nourish us and allow each partner to feel accepted, while unhealthy relationships cause harm because they involve trying to change your partner.

In an unhealthy relationship we unconsciously demand our partner to fulfil our needs for love and acceptance while simultaneously ignoring his or her needs. When both partners are trying to *get* what they need from, instead of *giving* to, their partner, conflict ensues.

Bad relationships are lacking in what both partners need. Our partners may *want* to give us what we need, but if they're struggling with low self-esteem they may simply be *unable* to, because they're also trying to get their own needs met, often in unhealthy and self-destructive ways.

If the arguments, frustration, lack of communication and stress continue, some relationships can become abusive. In you're in a relationship where either partner has lost the freedom to be themselves, to be independent and to remain in the relationship through choice rather than dependency, that relationship is destructive. If there is violence or physical or emotional abuse, leave the relationship and get professional help for yourself to help you recover and move forward. Remember that you deserve better.

Why do people with low self-esteem have unhealthy relationships?

We try to change our partner and find ourselves in a power struggle because we're trying to get our needs for love and acceptance met. These are basic human needs that were usually unmet during childhood. Children need to be loved, nurtured and to feel accepted for who they are. When these needs aren't met children become adults who continue to look for someone to fulfil this need and consequently become dependent on others to make them feel good about themselves. Understanding how your current relationships have been affected by your past can help you create real connections in the present.

In her book *Rewire Your Brain for Love*, the psychologist and neurologist Marsha Lucas explains that the first few years of life are a period of significant brain development, so our early experiences have a fundamental impact on our neural systems. Fearful events in childhood are imbedded into our brain and any fearful experience in subsequent relationships triggers that first experience – recalling the experience is the brain's way of trying to help you avoid being hurt again. But what helped you as a child doesn't often help as an adult.

Marilyn Sorensen, a clinical psychologist and self-esteem expert, suggests in her book *Breaking the Chain of Low Self-Esteem* that without the necessary support during our developmental years, some of us learn to avoid social situations and intimate relationships with others. Both dependent and avoidant types are unable to maintain healthy relationships and feel lonely and frustrated, but remain unable to change their lives.

Two psychology researchers, Sandra Murray and John Holmes, have developed the Risk Regulation Model to explain why people with low self-esteem tend to have relationships with more conflict and less love and trust. This model is based on three main concepts:

Concept 1 We all tend to assume other people see us in a similar way to how we see ourselves. People with low self-esteem tend to see themselves negatively and so doubt others will like them and whether their friends, family and partners will continue to love them and want them. Because their self-esteem depends on other people, their trust in others tends to fluctuate, depending on their mood or the circumstances.

Concept 2 People with low self-esteem tend to avoid complete commitment or intimacy because they find it difficult to believe they're unconditionally loved and accepted by their partners. This failure to allow themselves to become vulnerable, out of fear of being rejected, creates barriers between themselves and their loved ones.

Concept 3 People with low self-esteem have difficulty benefitting from the improved self-esteem healthy relationships can bring because they have trouble accepting their partner's positive view of them. If your partner sees you as smart, beautiful and talented, you'll tend to see those qualities in yourself over time. But if you have low self-esteem, you find it hard to believe those qualities are true.

In another study, these researchers found that people with low self-esteem dramatically underestimated how positively their partners saw them. These insecurities were associated with less positive perceptions of their partners and overall lower relationship well-being. Furthermore, the negative perceptions become worse over time, just as a positive perception became more reinforced over time.

How low self-esteem affects relationships

Staying in a bad relationship

While it's very difficult to end a love relationship, even when there's conflict, a situation in which there's constant struggle and frustration is not healthy for either partner. We end up feeling unloved, unheard and subjected to a lot of stress. Some people respond with rage, revenge or depression, or turn to drugs, alcohol, food or other addictions.

Many people find they can't leave such relationships, even when they know they're unhealthy. Remaining in this kind of relationship often creates so much stress that you're physically drained and lack the strength to leave. The damage it does to your self-esteem also tends to reinforce your belief that you don't deserve any better. You feel you can't leave because you're afraid you won't find anyone else. Many people in this situation also believe that if the relationship is not working, it's their fault. And so they continue to struggle and feel bad about themselves under the misguided belief that if only they try harder, they'll finally get the love they need.

This struggle to try harder lowers your self-esteem even further because your attempts to 'measure up' to fix the relationship are futile – you'll never be able to try hard enough to make things change. This is because the problem is not you – it's not your partner either. The problem is that you're both trying to get love and acceptance from each other while ignoring each other's needs. We can't get the love we need from someone who has nothing to give. If the relationship ends, we inevitably move on to another unhealthy relationship to look for love, and the cycle of struggle continues.

Testing a good relationship

Sometimes our low self-esteem causes us to test our relationships. If we don't feel we're truly deserving of love, we can feel confused and anxious when other people show love, respect and concern for us. At a subconscious level we don't believe it. Usually this is because our experience with love as children has been full of contradiction, such as parents throwing us birthday parties but never saying 'I love you'. Or perhaps the words were there but there were never hugs or cuddles. Or perhaps the message was consistently negative. This lack of certainty creates a sense of doubt in all our relationships and leaves us confused as to whom to trust and what to believe. All we know is that we don't feel loved or loveable, no matter what anyone says.

Marilyn Sorensen describes the way some people with low self-esteem test their relationships. They may create a set-up so that their friend or partner has to prove whether or not they really care about them. This usually happens subconsciously. For example, if you know your boyfriend has a football practice every Saturday morning, you might ask him to come shopping with you the following Saturday morning. If he changes his plans and comes with you, he has proved to you he loves you. Likewise, you might say nothing about your upcoming anniversary to see if your partner has remembered and planned something special, which would confirm he or she loves you. Any failure to pass these tests are automatically taken as signs of neglect, disinterest or a lack of caring.

There's usually a certain, specific outcome some people with low self-esteem have already created in their minds, and when this outcome comes to fruition, such as the boyfriend choosing shopping over football, they're satisfied and relieved that they're loved. But it's only temporary – they continue to worry about whether they're truly loved and accepted, and so will create another set-up. Nothing their partner does or says will be enough to convince them because they don't believe it themselves.

We test our relationships when we don't believe we're loved. We need evidence and proof that the love and friendship of others is genuine. Usually we don't realize we're testing our relationships, and in many cases are unable to see that it's inappropriate. We believe we're simply being cautious in knowing whom to trust. The person being tested is usually completely unaware of this test as well, until the tester becomes withdrawn, upset or angry when the desired outcome hasn't come about. We also don't realize we're sabotaging ourselves. In looking for continual reassurance that we're loved, we're placing our self-worth entirely in the hands of others and ignoring their needs and desires. With repetition this pattern can quickly erode the relationship, especially when the tested partner reacts to the tester with his or her own defensive, negative response.

The mindful way – living in the moment

Instead of attempting to fix our relationships by trying to change our partner, we need to change ourselves. This doesn't mean there's anything wrong with you or that everything is your fault. It means you're the only thing you *can* change. Fortunately, says Marsha Lucas, our brains are able to change – even as adults we're able to create new connections and new neurons and consequently new behaviours and ways of being.

'The most fundamental aggression to ourselves, the most fundamental harm we can do to ourselves,' says the Buddhist author Pema Chödrön in her book *When Things Fall Apart*, 'is to remain ignorant by not having the courage and the respect to look at ourselves honestly and gently.'

By focusing on you and your needs, at the present moment, you can learn to stop reacting to whatever your partner is doing or saying and simply be yourself, unaffected by the hurts of your past and unconcerned by worries or hopes about the future. When you're focused on the moment you can *choose* your actions consciously and wisely and in a state of calm, rational love, instead of unconscious, reactive fear.

> When Susan and Tom got into another argument, Susan became aware that she was feeling hurt and upset. She felt her mouth go dry and her hands begin to shake. Instead of running out of the room she decided to take a deep breath. She didn't say or do anything except breathe

slowly in and then out. Although Tom was clearly still angry, she felt calmer and then told him she felt hurt and upset. When he heard that, Tom realized he hadn't been aware of how much his reaction had upset her. He chose to listen to her and then he told her how he was feeling angry and criticized. It wasn't easy, but they were able to calm down and keep talking. Susan felt understood at last and Tom felt respected. And they were able to keep listening and give each other the love and acceptance they both needed.

Robin Norwood writes in her book *Women Who Love Too Much* that by being more focused on your own needs, you'll no longer need to seek security by trying to make others change. When you stop trying to get what you need from your partner, you can find it within yourself. It's there – you just have to believe it.

Once you believe you're loveable and deserving of love, you'll have love to give. Once you can give, you'll stop the struggle to get. You'll stop reacting out of fear that you won't get love. You'll choose to give. And you'll recognize that you deserve to be in a relationship in which both partners are loving and giving and both partners deserve love. You'll also start attracting partners who believe the same. When you're both giving, you'll both receive the love that's in you. You'll no longer be *reacting* because of the pain from the past but *acting* out of love in the moment.

Living in the moment means awareness in the moment

According to the mindfulness expert Jon Kabat-Zinn, mindfulness can help you focus on your needs in the moment because it's a process of bringing attention to moment-by-moment experience. By paying attention to your negative thoughts and feelings as they occur, you can learn to choose how to respond to them. Mindfulness gives us the choice to become present and aware in our lives or remain in a reactive, fearful state of 'autopilot'.

When we talk about living in the moment, says Ian Ellis Jones, a meditation specialist, we're concerned with being present and aware from one moment to the next. It's not existentially possible to live in the moment but it is possible to live fully aware. By becoming mindful, you become an observer of your thoughts as they occur instead of being a slave to them. Most of us are completely unaware of how much of our thinking is stuck in memories of past experiences or worries about the future, and until we focus on the present, they'll continue to affect our relationships now.

Awareness of your thoughts and feelings comes only by focusing on the here and now. Perhaps you've argued with your partner and you feel blamed. Your first reaction is that you want to get away. Acting on those impulses and running away, blaming, defending yourself or pushing those thoughts and feelings aside are reactions that only increase conflict. Instead, suggests the Buddhist teacher and clinical psychologist Tara Brach, pay attention to your thoughts and feelings – become aware of them; accept them. Stay in the present moment with whatever you're experiencing. You may find yourself feeling sad or angry or trapped, but by choosing to stay present rather than reacting, you can now choose how you want to respond. You can accept that those feelings are just feelings. It doesn't matter if you're angry, sad or annoyed, because those feelings are the *object* of your attention, not a reflection of who you are. You don't have to react to them to get the love you need. You can simply notice them and let them go and then deal with the argument calmly, rationally and focused on both your needs.

Being present in the moment is a choice

Choosing to be present means you're in control of how you act rather than your feelings and thoughts controlling you. By staying present and aware of your feelings you can choose to let them go. You can choose to be assertive and tell your partner how you're feeling and respond to his or her needs instead of escaping, blaming or defending yourself. This allows you to be more open and loving in your relationships instead of shutting down or shutting your partner out.

The result of choosing to be present rather than distant is an increase in your self-esteem. By choosing action over reaction you're telling yourself you deserve to live in love, not fear. It's this act of conscious choice that builds the foundation of our own self-worth, a foundation we create ourselves. Knowing you've chosen your own path means you're rejecting all the unkind, hurtful words and experiences of your past and are now creating a peaceful, loving experience in the present. By taking responsibility for your own happiness and getting your own needs met in this way, you're developing your self-esteem, moment by moment.

Mindful practices to keep you in the moment

Breathing

Focusing on your breathing is the best and simplest way to bring yourself back from the past and the future to the present moment. When you pay attention to your body you'll notice the way it responds to stress and strong emotions. You may notice your heart pounding, your hands sweating, a feeling of dizziness. These physical responses are your body's reactions to your fears about the future or your worries about the past. When you become aware of these reactions in your body, it's a signal that you need to bring yourself back to the present moment. The best way to do this is with breathing. Take a deep breath and think about only your inhalation and then your exhalation. This will calm your fears and anxieties, lower your heart rate and keep you focused on your present experience. In the words of the mindfulness expert Thich Nhat Hanh, 'Feelings come and go like clouds in a windy sky. Conscious breathing is my anchor.'

Savouring

Savouring is the term psychologists use to describe the experience of appreciating or luxuriating in whatever you're doing at the present moment. Whether you're eating an apple, taking a shower or walking to the bus stop, savouring usually involves your senses. In a study by the psychologist Stephen Schueller, when participants took a few minutes each day to savour something they usually hurried through, they began to experience more joy, happiness and other positive emotions and fewer depressive symptoms. When we learn to savour our experiences we become less focused on our negative thoughts and worries and more on living in the present.

Pausing

In her book mentioned earlier in this chapter, Marsha Lucas suggests pausing for six seconds periodically throughout the day – you can take a pause every hour or every time you make a cup of tea, for example. This helps you to slow down and turn off your autopilot and focus on the present moment. It also resets your nervous system so you can choose how to respond instead of reacting.

Silence

Whenever you're practising mindfulness you're enjoying silence. You stop the talking outside but also the talking inside your mind. The talking inside is the thinking that goes on and on and often creates unpleasant feelings. Mindfulness is not the kind of silence that oppresses us, says Thich Nhat Hanh; it's the kind that heals and nourishes us.

Meditation

According to recent research, mindfulness meditation can help you focus on the moment. A study published in the journal *NeuroReport* found that experienced meditators had an increased thickness in the brain regions associated with attention and sensory processing. Likewise, a study in *Frontiers in Human Neuroscience* found that long-time meditators increased folding of the cortex, which scientists believe helps the brain process information faster and appears to be involved in emotion regulation and self-awareness. According to the psychiatrist Daniel Siegel, even as little as three minutes of mindfulness meditation a day can change your brain. Marsha Lucas says that the brain seems to benefit more from frequent, short meditations than less frequent, longer ones.

Repeat

A daily meditation practice can build your mindfulness muscle the same way regular exercise builds your body's muscles. With repeated practice you'll grow stronger over time. One meditation technique is called walking meditation. You simply walk and enjoy every step, fully present in the here and now. When you walk like that, says Thich Nhat Hanh, every step brings healing.

It's important to keep practising mindfulness, by breathing, meditating, bringing your focus to the present moment and choosing the way you want to respond. Joseph Burgo, the author of *Why Do I Do That?*, agrees:

You'll never arrive at the 'new and improved' you who no longer needs to struggle. As you go, you'll continue to face additional challenges, feeling a pull to cope with them in the old familiar ways. As a result, you'll confront one choice after another – to go with your defences or try to cope in a different way. If you maintain the mindset for change and choose well, at least some of the time, you will continue to grow throughout your life.

Every time you react with frustration, sadness or anger, says Jon Kabat-Zinn, you're practising mind*less*ness. Every time you react you're reinforcing your own negative thoughts and beliefs, activating your fears and becoming better at reacting. You're creating a habit of not paying attention and ignoring your own needs as well as the needs and feelings of others. Mindfulness practice helps you to break that habit and stop reacting in a negative way. With practice, you're developing a presence of mind that will be able to deal with difficult situations as they arise and free you to make the choices that are right for you.

3

Defensiveness or awareness

By transforming our unconscious behaviour into a conscious behaviour – that is, by becoming aware of it – we can take back control of our actions and choose the way we want to respond.

Tom and Susan often found themselves arguing over small things. The arguments would escalate until Susan left the room and Tom was slamming doors. Neither of them could understand why things always got so heated.

'I just want to know why you got home late and didn't call me,' said Susan. 'I had dinner waiting and now it's ruined.'

'And I suppose that's all my fault?' Tom replied. 'You always blame me for everything. Well, what about the time you stayed late at your sister's and didn't call me?'

'What's that have to do with anything?'

'It has everything to do with it because I'm not the one at fault here. I didn't do anything wrong!'

What is defensiveness?

Defensiveness is a common reaction that leads to communication problems in relationships. Defensiveness is harmful because it puts us in a closed-minded, self-protective mode. We can't listen to other people's points of view or appreciate how they're feeling. It usually triggers them to respond with anger, frustration or their own defensiveness, creating further conflict and leaving both parties feeling misunderstood, hurt and resentful. It also pushes other people away and creates barriers to love and intimacy, which are the very things we're seeking.

We all have a need to feel competent, appreciated, valued and loved. We want to feel we're smart, capable and loveable. When someone shares their concerns or points out our mistakes, people with low self-esteem can feel criticized or attacked, and often respond by getting defensive, whether the other person intended to criticize or not. We try to explain our actions, justify our behaviour and deflect responsibility away from ourselves by pointing the finger at someone else.

Most of the time we're not even aware we're acting this way, but our own defensiveness can quickly trigger defensiveness, anger and resentment in the other person. Defensiveness is an understandable attempt to protect ourselves, but it isn't very effective. It destroys our relationships by eroding communication and damages our self-esteem by keeping us trapped in a state of fear.

We all want to be accepted and loved for who we are. So if you feel there's something wrong with you, when someone says something that sounds like it might be a criticism or complaint about you, it's just too painful to hear. What's left is a dangerously fragile person who hears every word, every encounter, as a personal attack and comes out fighting to try to avoid getting hurt again. You live in a state of constant vigilance against possible threats to your emotional well-being. Instead of listening you start explaining, and instead of communicating you start avoiding, all of which are sure ways of escalating conflict in your relationships.

According to the relationship expert John Gottman, defensiveness backfires because it's really a way of blaming partners. When we're defensive we're saying, 'The problem isn't me, it's you.' Whether they meant to criticize us or not, they rarely back down but instead try harder to get us to see their point of view. And ultimately the defender ends up hurting others and pushing people away – the very result that was most feared.

What causes defensiveness?

Feeling criticized or attacked is actually only the trigger for a defensive reaction. The real cause is a deep feeling of inadequacy. If we've been judged, blamed, criticized or controlled as a child, we inevitably grow up feeling there's something wrong with us. We feel we're not good enough. Consequently, says Joseph Burgo, the author of *Why Do I Do That?*, instead of developing the self-confidence that's built on trust, we feel a deep sense of shame.

The shame that results from being let down by our parents fills us with the belief that we're unlovable. According to Burgo, people who struggle with shame often respond with blaming, contempt and narcissism. They have a hard time acknowledging their own faults or errors and blame others, thereby projecting what they perceive to be their own inner ugliness onto other people. They don't recognize their defensiveness because their attention is consistently focused on someone else.

Once those negative thoughts and beliefs become planted in us when we're young, they tend to stay with us, becoming further embedded in our sense of self with every conversation. The defence mechanisms we develop growing up were useful then and usually helped us to survive at a time when we were most vulnerable. But the strategies we used as children now serve only to weaken us, blocking our engagement with and intimate connection to our partners. We become anxious and jealous, fearing our partner will find out our defects and reject us.

Why is it difficult to change?

Increasingly our subconscious minds seek out people and situations that reinforce our negative beliefs because we're attracted to what's familiar to us, whether it's positive or negative. At the same time, these experiences only serve to bring us more pain and we react in the only way we know how, by getting defensive and once again reinforcing the idea in our own minds that we're inadequate.

Low self-esteem often provokes feelings of anxiety and fear because we're constantly on the lookout for signs of danger, which can be anything from a co-worker's snub to the tone in our partner's voice. When we sense that a criticism, judgement, complaint or attack is coming, our defences are triggered. This is a subconscious process and most of us are unaware of our own defensive behaviour. It's the mind's way of trying to protect us from harm, but defences are really only tactics to avoid facing reality. In effect they're a way of distancing ourselves from an awareness of unpleasant thoughts, feelings and behaviours. This avoidance provides a short-term relief for our fears and anxieties but our defences inevitably rise again with the next encounter, creating more distance between ourselves and the people we love.

According to Susan Johnson, a research expert on intimacy, the drive to survive and restore our sense of safety subconsciously overrides our drive for love. Consequently we say things and do things to protect ourselves, even when it sabotages our own happiness. When our subconscious minds sense danger, for example in the form of harmless criticism, concern or a complaint, we tend to seek safety by creating distance between ourselves and others, both physically and emotionally. In this way, we create the very situation we're attempting to avoid, which is pushing other people away and avoiding the intimacy, connection and love we crave.

Types of defences

Sigmund Freud began writing about psychological defences in the 1890s. He believed that when we're confronted with a feeling we find too painful we automatically push it into our subconscious mind where we don't have to think about it. Anna Freud continued her father's work by defining the different types of defence mechanisms:

- *Denial* – claiming/believing that what is true is actually false.
- *Displacement* – redirecting emotions to a substitute target.
- *Intellectualization* – taking an objective viewpoint and avoiding emotions.
- *Projection* – attributing uncomfortable feelings to others and assuming others are reacting to you as disapprovingly as you are.
- *Rationalization* – creating false but credible justifications.
- *Reaction formation* – expressing the opposite of your feelings in your behaviour.
- *Regression* – reverting to acting as a child.
- *Repression* – pushing uncomfortable thoughts into the subconscious.
- *Sublimation* – redirecting 'wrong' urges into socially acceptable actions.

There are several ways these mechanisms translate into our everyday behaviours and responses. In his book *Why Marriages Succeed or Fail*, John Gottman describes seven common signs of defensiveness:

1 *Making excuses* This tactic involves explaining your actions and justifying your behaviour based on the claim that external forces beyond your control forced you to act in a certain way. For example, when your wife asks you why you didn't call to say you'd be late, you tell her your phone battery died and you were rushing to get home. In this way you blame everything but yourself and refuse to take any responsibility for your actions.

2 *Cross-complaining* When your partner complains or criticizes, you immediately respond with a complaint or criticism of your own. You ignore what your partner has said and go on the attack.

3 *Table turning* Instead of listening, we blame our partner for the same thing he or she is criticizing us about. If, for example, when you're late home from work your partner tells you the dinner has gone cold, and you respond by saying you had to wait for her at the store on the weekend and missed your football game, you're using the past as a weapon to cope with the present.

4 *Yes-butting* This means starting sentences with agreement and ending them with disagreement to justify your position. This response is an attempt to placate your partner while explaining you're not at fault and you deserve more sympathy. Once again, this places all the responsibility on your partner instead of you, and allows you to avoid dealing with his or her feelings.

5 *Repeating* When you think you're right and your partner is wrong, you repeat your point of view increasingly louder and more forcefully and ignore your partner's. This can also include talking incessantly so your partner doesn't have a chance to express opinions or feelings and therefore can't criticize you.

6 *Denying responsibility* Avoiding responsibility for your behaviour is a key facet of all defensive behaviour. You insist you're not to blame, no matter what your partner says or how guilty you actually are, as a way of avoiding perceived criticism.

7 *Tone and body language* We can say a lot without using words. Standing with our arms crossed, rolling our eyes, smirking, laughing or ignoring our partner are just some of the ways we try to defend ourselves and avoid facing our partner's thoughts and feelings.

No matter how we express our low self-esteem, our defensive behaviours are inherently an automatic response to what we believe to be a criticism or attack on us. Automatic responses are subconscious, meaning we're usually unaware of them and also that they're triggered by a deep-rooted survival instinct that doesn't involve our conscious, rational mind. Our ability to think clearly is turned off and we enter a 'fight or flight' response to what we believe is a threat.

In this way we're motivated by fear rather than love, and living in a state of *reaction* rather than *action*. What this means is that our sense of safety and well-being is left in the hands of others and changes according to what is said or done to us, because we haven't learned how to create our own sense of inner safety.

According to Susan Johnson, reacting is a blame pattern of thinking, and a mindset of blame leaves us feeling powerless, which weakens our self-esteem. Reacting defensively causes us to think that we can't be happy or feel loved, valued or deserving unless someone else does or says something a certain way. This in turn leads us to focus our efforts on changing or controlling the thoughts, feelings and behaviours of others rather than ourselves. Since we can't control others we're left feeling even more powerless, anxious and insecure, along with any number of other emotions, including anger, resentment, depression and bitterness.

The mindful way   awareness

Instead of defending ourselves, blaming others, avoiding responsibility and surrendering our sense of safety to other people and external circumstances, we need to find the courage to face our fears and remain emotionally present. When we feel we're in danger, especially in the form of what we imagine will be criticism about who we are or a judgement about whether or not we're adequate and loveable, we react in ways that sabotage our own happiness. We react negatively because we're driven by fear. By developing awareness we can stay connected to our loved ones and experience the acceptance, understanding and love we're longing for.

Awareness means allowing yourself to feel those deep-rooted fears of being judged, blamed, criticized, dismissed and rejected, and *not* letting fear trigger your response. It's not easy to stop defending your-self when you've been reacting this way for a long time, particularly because it's an *unconscious* behaviour. But by transforming it into a *conscious* behaviour – that is, by becoming aware of it – we can take back control of our actions and choose the way we want to respond.

Mindfulness is being aware of what is happening in the present moment without judging it or trying to change it. This is an impor-tant tool for overcoming low self-esteem because the defensive tactics we use to try to change a situation only serve to weaken our self-esteem. When we act defensively we live in a state of constant struggle, always on the alert for possible threats to our confidence, always quickly rising to defend ourselves against these threats, always trying to prove ourselves worthy.

Defence mechanisms are an attempt to convert reality as it is into a version we find acceptable. Mindfulness encourages us to accept reality in the present moment. Awareness is a vital part of growing our self-esteem because it encourages us to stop struggling and see things as they are.

During arguments with partners, for example, awareness allows us to see that their concerns are about their own real, unmet needs, not an attack on us. Their concerns are often just the trigger for our own fears. With this awareness we can recognize how we're responding and when and how we're becoming defensive. In this way mindfulness boosts our awareness of how we're interpreting and reacting to our own fears. By becoming more aware we can create a moment between our emotions and our actions. We can then use that moment to choose to respond in a healthier way rather than simply reacting to an imagined threat. It's what Buddhists call recognizing the spark before the flame.

In a study by Sean Barnes and colleagues in the *Journal of Marital and Family Therapy*, researchers showed that instead of just helping people cope with the effects of emotional reactions during personal conflict, mindfulness prevents them rising to a defensive reaction. The study also showed that mindfulness enabled people to be more present with their partner when they're in a situation that could provoke a defence.

By becoming mindfully aware we can notice how our thoughts and feelings can change our perception of reality and allow us to pay attention to our own responses and how those responses affect others. We can learn to listen without fear, act instead of react and accept others' thoughts, feelings and even criticism without defensiveness. This awareness allows us to choose to let go of old habits and reduce their power to influence us. And it builds our self-esteem because we're taking responsibility for our own thoughts, feelings and behaviour instead of living life trying to defend ourselves.

Developing awareness of our thoughts, feelings and reactions doesn't mean we're trying to get rid of them. It simply means we're moving out of a subconscious, fear-based, fight-or-flight reaction and into a conscious recognition of how we're feeling and thinking in a particular moment. Any time we're reacting out of fear, we're in a victim role. When our thoughts and behaviour repeat themselves it's easy to become locked in this role and we then identify ourselves with this concept of who we are. When we continue to react out of fear, our thoughts and actions reinforce this concept, thereby lowering our self-esteem. We believe this is who we are and then we live according to this identity, seeking out people and experiences that perpetuate it and ignoring or rejecting anything to the contrary.

By becoming aware of ourselves we can begin to see that thoughts and feelings and even our own self-concept aren't set in stone but are temporary and changeable. We can change them. By developing awareness we can stop avoiding the thoughts and feelings that frighten us. Avoidance only creates further feelings of shame and self-criticism. Instead we can face the fear, the painful memories and the hurt feelings that have kept us trapped. We can simply accept them as the transient objects they are rather than fixed aspects of who we are. In this way we can take control of how we respond and who we choose to be. We can begin to choose to live the life we want – one of peace and calm, happiness and love.

Once we develop an awareness of how we're reacting to our own fears and to other people, we'll start to let go of our defensiveness and communicate more effectively.

'I want to know why you're home late and didn't call me,' said Susan in an anxious tone. 'I had dinner waiting and now it's ruined.'

'It wasn't my fault,' Tom replied. 'My meeting ran late and I couldn't get out of it.'

Susan took a deep breath. 'I'm not blaming you. I just wanted you to call me. I felt anxious.'

Tom stopped talking for a moment. He could hear how defensive he was sounding. He felt his heart pounding and he knew he was feeling attacked. He took a deep breath, let go of his fear of being blamed and focused on what his wife was saying. 'You must have been worried,' he said.

'Yes I was,' Susan replied, sounding calmer. 'And I feel frustrated that the dinner is ruined.'

'I understand.' Tom took her hand and looked at her. 'That would be frustrating.'

'Thank you.' Susan took a deep breath. 'Will you ring me next time?'

'I will.' Tom smiled. 'How about we order Chinese takeaway tonight?'

'Good idea!'

How to develop awareness

The key to developing mindful awareness is to practise it, both in the moment and as a daily exercise. You can begin to become more aware of your defensive reactions by listening to your body. When we feel threatened our central nervous system responds by preparing us physically to either fight or flee. Even if the threat is the voice of your partner rather than an approaching tiger, your brain and your body respond the same way.

When you feel stressed your body releases stress hormones, such as cortisol, to boost your blood sugar levels to give you energy. Your heart rate quickens and you can experience an array of sensations including dizziness, dry mouth, headache, muscle tension, shortness of breath, sweating and trembling. In addition, fear can make you feel edgy and irritable, unable to concentrate, panicked or upset, causing you to seek reassurance desperately from others or go on the attack. Your brain goes into survival mode and you start operating on instinct rather than rational thought, which is why we say things we later regret, fail to listen properly and hurt the ones we love. This in turn lowers our self-esteem even further.

These symptoms are signs your body is preparing for action. But by becoming aware of them we can recognize the moment we're slipping into a reactive, defensive mode and can choose an alternative.

The following mindfulness exercises can help you to become more aware of your body and your mind and the ways you respond to stress. Once you're aware of what you're doing and how you're feeling, you can choose how to respond:

Breathing

One of the best ways of becoming more aware is simply breathing. Mindful deep breathing can reduce anxiety and raise the levels of hormones in the brain – such as oxytocin and dopamine – that make you feel good, and lower cortisol, the hormone released by stress. When you breathe deeply you experience better mental clarity, focus, attention and concentration.

The Zen master and spiritual leader Thich Nhat Hanh suggests taking a deep breath and slowly exhaling while you think to yourself, 'Breathing in, I'm aware of my body. Breathing out, I release the tension in my body.'

Breathing also makes you more aware of your body. When you're aware of your body you're centred in the present moment. Simply become aware of the breath you're breathing in and out. By focusing on your breathing in this way, the noise of your thoughts disappears. Your mind will calm because your attention is focused on your breathing. Your heart rate will slow down and you'll be able to focus on the moment, instead of the fears that well up from the past or the anxieties created about the future. Once you're focused on the moment you'll be able to focus on what your partner is saying rather than trying to predict or control his or her thoughts and behaviour.

Journalling

The psychologist and mindfulness author Elisha Goldstein suggests writing down your thoughts and feelings in a mindfulness journal. When faced with negative judgements or self-criticisms, writing them down can separate those thoughts from the emotions and self-perceptions we attach to them. It also helps us to become aware of what we're thinking and feeling, which is crucial because many of our thoughts and feelings are locked in our subconscious mind and writing can help to bring them into our awareness. This also helps us to avoid thinking obsessively about the negative feelings and thoughts – writing gets it down on paper and out of our minds.

Like any practice, such as playing the piano or exercise, the more you practise mindfulness the better you become. Practising a daily mindfulness exercise can help to keep you calm and focused on the moment and develop your awareness. Try five minutes of focused breathing every day – when you're not feeling stressed – as a regular practice and you'll begin to become more aware of your body, your thoughts, feelings and your responses.

4

Control or acceptance

Acceptance doesn't mean you play the victim and simply accept others' treatment of you. It means you accept yourself as you are, with all your faults and failings and all your positive qualities.

Susan had been married to Tom for 15 years. When they first started dating, she'd found him fun and exciting and he'd made her happy. But over the years, she found she was having to try harder and harder to please him. He had a certain way he liked her to do things, but it seemed no matter how hard she tried, nothing she did was ever good enough. She believed that if she was failing everyone, she must not be good enough. She knew there must be something wrong with her.

What is controlling behaviour?

Low self-esteem is a basic tendency to place your value in the hands of others rather than trusting and believing in your own evaluation of yourself. If your self-esteem depends on other people's view of you, it becomes fragile and unstable, fluctuating daily with your experiences and the opinions of other people. Consequently people with low self-esteem often feel a sense of having no control over their lives. They tend to cope with this feeling of powerlessness either by allowing other people to control them or by trying to regain their power by controlling everyone around them.

A person with healthy self-esteem still cares what other people think but they don't let others' opinions or judgements form the basis of their feelings about themselves. They assume that what they do, what they say and who they are is all right with others, and their behaviour is a reflection of their belief that they're acceptable.

Normal human behaviour includes the desire to have some control over our lives and our surroundings. It gives us a sense of stability, predictability and safety. Desiring control over oneself is a healthy aspect of controlling behaviour. Likewise, there's also a need to exert some control over your children's behaviour or students in a classroom. But when you're driven to control others it's usually based on fear and usually leads to the decline of your relationships as well as your own and others' self-esteem.

A number of strategies may be used to control yourself or others. Many of the tactics a person uses are repeated from childhood experiences with a controlling parent, and may include:

- anger and aggression
- acting like a victim or a martyr
- restricting a partner's freedoms
- controlling finances
- using religion to make someone feel guilty
- belittling and criticizing
- threatening to end the relationship
- passive-aggression, such as pretending to be nice to create a sense of obligation
- silent treatment
- expecting mind-reading
- dominating conversations
- asking for an opinion and then responding to the answer as if it were a personal attack
- correcting others
- changing the subject
- enforcing a double standard
- constantly raising the bar
- intimidation, threats, bullying
- lying
- violating others' personal boundaries
- constant talking to avoid the possible criticisms of others.

While they may appear needy and incapable, says Joseph Burgo, the author of *Why Do I Do That?*, some people with low self-esteem have an unacknowledged hope of controlling their partners. Through their helpless behaviour they're forcing the other person to assume the role of caretaker and they can then manipulate the partner into giving what is wanted, be it emotional or financial support.

What causes controlling behaviour?

Growing up with a controlling parent is one of the main reasons for controlling behaviour in relationships. According to Rick Fitzgibbons, the director of the Institute for Marital Healing in Philadelphia, people can resort to controlling behaviours because they feel a lack of trust with their partner, which stems from a lack of trust with their parent.

Another source of controlling behaviour is a stressful and/or traumatic childhood involving abandonment, abuse, or a parent with an addiction or an angry or narcissistic personality. In some cases controlling people are also narcissistic and simply insist on being in control.

For most people the pain of trying to cope with a controlling parent is very difficult to face and many will project either their own emotional pain onto someone else or accuse their partner of being the controller. A controlling parent can also lead some people to fear being controlled as an adult, which often results in behaviour intended to keep others at an emotional distance. Sometimes there can be a confusing mixture of behaviours, when people who have been controlled push loved ones away out of fear of being controlled and then pull them closer again out of need for approval.

Are you being controlled?

Some people respond to this feeling of lack of empowerment by continuing to allow others to control them. Most often they're completely unaware it's happening or why. When someone controls you, however, your ability to say and do what you think and feel is right is limited. Your ability to develop as a person and be who you really are is restricted. As the controlling behaviour continues, the controller creates insecurity and dependency in you and you end up ignoring and discounting your own thoughts, feelings, needs and your sense of self.

If you believe other people have control over you, a controlling person may feel, on a subconscious level, like a relief to you because he or she will be doing exactly what you expect people to do; that is, control you. They'll probably make you feel very comfortable, at least at first. Most people who are controlled by others have usually had similar experiences in childhood. When you're raised by a controlling person this kind of behaviour seems natural to you. It feels familiar and therefore safe. You cling to it because your mind registers this behaviour as 'normal' for you.

As you grow up you're influenced not only by your genetic makeup but by the behaviour of the people closest to you. In many cases, if one of your parents had a controlling nature, the other parent was probably more submissive. Consequently some people will identify with and model the behaviour of the passive parent so that they become attracted to a controlling partner and assume the submissive role in their own relationships, just as their parent did.

Unfortunately your attraction to what's familiar to you is not necessarily what's good for you. Engaging in any kind of relationship with someone who seeks to control you will reinforce your belief that it's all right and you don't deserve any better. The longer you remain in these kinds of relationships, the more they erode your sense of self-worth, plunging your self-esteem into a downward spiral in which you increasingly seek the reassurance of controlling people to make you feel good about yourself – the very people whose behaviour is exacerbating your low self-esteem.

Are you controlling?

Some people have grown up with a controlling parent and model that parent's behaviour by being controlling themselves. They may try to regain a sense of control in their lives by controlling other people. In some cases they may have been neglected or abused, leaving them with an uncontrollable anger with which they lash out, or they may use strategies to control others emotionally.

People who are controlling often appear to be confident and assertive, but it's a cover for their own deep-rooted feelings of insecurity. At the heart of controlling behaviour is a feeling of shame; they're ashamed of who they are because they believe – or have been led to believe – that they're not good enough. Consequently they believe that an authoritative manner will keep other people in line and allow them to feel more in control and therefore better about themselves. By putting others down they can build themselves up. This kind of controlling behaviour also includes passive-aggressive techniques, such as always being late or refusing to take responsibility for anything. In this way they can get what they want through manipulation.

According to the psychologist Les Parrott, author of *The Control Freak*, controlling people operate under the mistaken belief that what they can control can't hurt them. Driven by the fear that their own flaws and vulnerabilities will become exposed and used against them, they try to hide behind a dominating persona and control every aspect of their environment and the people in it. Like anyone with low self-esteem, their sense of self-worth is entirely dependent on the approval of others, which is why they work so hard to appear to be in control. They need the approval of others while at the same time refusing to trust anyone, fearing any sign of weakness will mean being at the mercy of others.

Unfortunately this approach inevitably backfires because other people increasingly disapprove of their controlling behaviour. Their self-esteem sinks even further, leading them to behave in ever more controlling ways in a desperate attempt to feel worthy. The more they try to control people and events the more frustrated, angry and powerless they end up feeling.

Are men and women different?

Men and women can often exhibit control issues differently. Men will usually try to control others as a way of coping with their own insecurities. They tend to use abusive and bullying tactics to dominate others and transfer their own emotional pain onto other people. The more they can control the people they love, the more in control and powerful they feel. For a controlling man this is the best way to avoid feeling weak, which is unbearable for him.

Women who have been victims of bullying or abuse, neglect or abandonment may use control tactics to regain a sense of control over their lives. Women who had alcoholic fathers are particularly susceptible to becoming controlling themselves as a way of coping with the lack of control in their childhood. Women's control issues tend to emerge as food, shopping or alcohol addictions, jealousy, overprotectiveness, anxiety or self-harm.

When people with control issues experience a difficult event (such as job loss, losing a loved one or a relationship break-up), feel they've failed or are being blamed, or any time they feel emotionally vulnerable, their control issues may be enhanced as they attempt to recover their sense of self.

It's important to remember that none of this is your fault. Neither your upbringing nor your parents' behaviour nor even its consequences are your fault. At the same time it's important not to blame your parents – they had their faults and struggles and probably tried their best. The key to changing the unhealthy control issues in your life now is to recognize there's nothing wrong with you, just as you are. If control issues have become part of your life, whether because other people tend to control you or you find yourself controlling them, you can live a more balanced, peaceful life where the only control you have is over your own life.

The mindful way – acceptance

Mindfulness encourages you to see things as they are now and accept them. Acknowledging and accepting your feelings, your beliefs, your behaviour, instead of denying them, puts you in a more powerful position because you can do something about them. It puts you in control of your life instead of allowing fear or the feelings from the past to control you.

The next step is to recognize that you have a choice. You can choose to continue in the same way you always have, choosing people and situations that feel familiar and comfortable for you but ultimately make you feel bad about yourself and lower your self-esteem because they reinforce your negative beliefs. Or you can choose a different approach. We all choose certain options and behave in certain ways because of the way we feel about ourselves. Once you're aware of those beliefs and the way they drive you to make unhealthy choices, you can choose to hang on to them or let them go.

> Tom had always known Susan loved him and would do anything for him. The problem was that his sense of self-worth depended on this. If Susan was compliant he felt loved; if she wasn't he felt ignored and

unloved. Over time this pattern meant Susan had to keep doing more and more to satisfy Tom's need for love, though it was a need only he could fill.

When she came home from work that night, Susan knew Tom was expecting to discuss something with her. She was worried because she was exhausted and wanted to say no, but knew if she did she'd feel she was letting him down and being selfish.

'We need to talk about the vacation plans I've made after dinner,' Tom said without even looking at her.

Susan smiled, happy he wanted to do so much for her. But then she became aware that she felt sad, that she didn't feel loved and that she'd always done things for others but still felt she wasn't good enough, recognizing that feeling from when she was growing up. It scared her to say no but she didn't want to be controlled any more.

'Can we talk about it over the weekend?' she said nervously. 'I'm tired and just want to relax this evening, but I'd like to discuss the plans so we can decide together.'

'Oh – that's not like you. I thought you liked me taking control of things.'

'I know. I did. It feels a bit scary to change – but it makes me feel good about myself to tell you what I want.'

'Okay. So this isn't about me doing a bad job, is it?'

'No. You're doing a great job. It's about me. I just want to feel more like an equal partner.'

'Okay – I just want you to be happy.' Tom smiled. By giving up control he realized he felt nervous too, but better, happier, easier. Now he didn't have to do it all alone – they could do this together.

What is acceptance?

Acceptance is a fundamental part of mindfulness. Acceptance doesn't mean you play the victim and simply accept others' treatment of you. It means you accept yourself as you are, with all your faults and failings and all your positive qualities. You accept the world as it is, with parents who may have let you down and partners who may be more interested in their own self-esteem issues than in you. You can accept these things while knowing that none of it changes the fact that you're all right just as you are. You're lovable and deserve to be loved.

Recognizing where your negative beliefs came from and the feelings associated with them is crucial. According to Rick Fitzgibbons, without uncovering the anger, resentment and hurt you feel towards a controlling parent, you'll remain stuck emotionally in the past. The fear of getting hurt again will control your future relationships by driving you to repeat that controlling behaviour with your partner as well as misdirecting your rage and resentment for your parent at your partner.

Mindful acceptance means that once you become aware of what is driving your behaviour you focus your attention on what is happening now, with the people who are here with you now. Allowing your attention to wander can leave you feeling anxious about what happened in the past or worried about what might happen in the future. Acceptance means staying present and seeing the present moment as it is, without needing to control anyone or feeling fear or anger or denial. It is without criticism or judgement or blame. It just is.

Staying in the present can be challenging because it can feel uncomfortable. If you've had negative beliefs about yourself for a long time it can feel strange to let them go, as if you're shedding your skin. It feels new and strange and you can feel very exposed and vulnerable without that wall of resentment and avoidance you've built around yourself. It can feel awkward to let go of the anger and hurt you've held on to for so long. It can feel frightening to accept yourself as you are and to believe you're acceptable. But resisting that acceptance, fighting against it, struggling to hold on to the past – even a painful past – is what creates stress, damages relationships and erodes self-esteem. Letting go of your attempts to control others or of allowing them to control you, and accepting the past for what it is – namely the past – increases your self-esteem.

Accept yourself

Choosing acceptance allows you to accept yourself and love yourself, instead of relying on other people to determine your worth. In this way it doesn't matter what anyone says or does, what your parents told you or how your partner criticizes you – you've chosen to accept yourself. That's when healthy self-esteem is born. It means you don't need other people to tell you what to do, what to think, how to behave or how to run your life so that you're constantly struggling to do the right thing. It means you don't need other people to tell you who you are or what you are because you already know. You know you're loveable.

Trying to fulfil others' demands of you all the time will only make you feel that nothing you do is good enough – there'll always be something you haven't done well or fast enough; always something else for you to do because this keeps those others in control. They don't ever want you to do a good enough job, but to keep struggling because that keeps you needing their approval. But all you need to feel good about yourself is your own approval and your own acceptance.

Let go of control

Mindful acceptance also allows you to let go of controlling others when you accept yourself as a worthy person and accept others as they are. In his book *Wise Mind, Open Mind*, Ronald Alexander explains the eightfold path developed by Buddha, which is a way of looking at the world in a mindful way. The first path is called wise view, which is recognizing that it's not in your power to control what happens outside of you. You can only control what happens in your own mind.

Fear that other people will control you and the belief that they'll judge you as harshly as you judge yourself keeps you trapped in a damaging cycle of denial, repression and dependence on others' submission to feel good about yourself. The problem with this approach is that it's like an addiction: there's a short-term boost when you manipulate someone into doing what you want but it doesn't last long. Your self-esteem actually takes a hit from such hurtful behaviour because you're repeating the painful experiences of your past and reinforcing the belief that you're not good enough. You have to try harder, become more demanding and controlling, to try to feel good again. Holding on to painful feelings also takes a toll on your health because your body's stress-response system is activated by this imagined threat.

Mindfulness also provides the clarity and focus that allows you to see your own behaviour and the damaging way you're trying to control your life by controlling others. With acceptance, you see that control hurts others and weakens your own self-esteem because you're not in control of yourself.

Forgive

Breaking this cycle of fear, anger and control requires acceptance and forgiveness. The only way you can let go of the anger and hurt you feel towards your controlling parent is to acknowledge it and forgive. Painful feelings simply don't go away on their own, no matter how much we try to avoid them, deny them, bury them and blame other people for them. Such tactics usually make the feelings grow because you're focusing your energy on resisting them.

If you're fighting, you have to have something to fight against; stop fighting, stop resisting, and the enemy disappears. You're trying to keep fear, pain, criticism, rejection at bay because you believe they'll hurt you. But that pain comes from the past. Facing it, accepting it, forgiving those who hurt you will disarm it so you can turn your attention to the present moment, where you can choose who you are, what you want and what you believe about yourself. According to the forgiveness researcher Sam Standard (Harris et al., 2006), mindfulness mind–body practices allow you literally to feel how not forgiving is affecting you and to become open to positive alternatives.

Arnie Kozak, a mindfulness-based psychotherapist, suggests that forgiveness can be a private process of acceptance. It doesn't have to involve the people who've upset you. It's not about demanding an apology or evoking guilt. It's not about condoning their behaviour or telling yourself that what they did or said was in order. It's about not letting the past control how you feel or how you behave in the present.

5

Perfectionism or non-judgement

Acceptance is what dissolves the anxiety, the fear and the need to keep trying to win approval. Accepting yourself without judgement means you already have that approval.

Susan's mother was coming for dinner and she wanted everything to be perfect. Growing up, she'd always felt she wasn't good enough because her mother had criticized her for being too skinny and too shy. Even as an adult she felt her mouth go dry and her voice start to quiver when her mother questioned her cooking or her choice of clothes. Tom had offered to clean up the garden and wash the car but when he was finished, Susan pointed out the spots he'd missed and complained that he'd done a bad job. He said he was sorry but Susan stormed off. When he went into the kitchen he found her vacuuming inside the kitchen cupboards.

'What are you doing?' Tom asked. 'Your mother's not going to look in there. She's only coming for dinner.'

'Look at this! There are crumbs in here. This isn't good enough.'

'Let me help you.'

'No, I'll do it. If I don't, she'll know. She'll know I've let it slip. Oh, why is this place such a mess? Why can't I do anything right?'

What is perfectionism?

While low self-esteem can manifest itself outwardly as fearfulness or timidity, it can also present as over-achievement. People with low self-esteem tend to compare themselves with others and consequently may set very high goals or become overly competitive in an attempt to boost their sense of self-worth. They may also become perfectionists, living with the belief that nothing they do or achieve is ever good enough. They keep trying to gain what they believe will be others' acceptance, but live with a constant feeling of failure and inadequacy.

As Joseph Burgo explains in *Why Do I Do That?*, people with low self-esteem expect themselves to be perfect to escape from and disprove their sense of worthlessness. When they fail to meet their own high standards they feel so much self-loathing that they often turn the blame on others. This not only alienates them from other people but also means they don't learn from their experiences because they believe the fault lies with someone else.

These attempts to reach a state of perfection are harmful because nothing is ever enough. By constantly struggling to reach an unrealistic goal or status we're holding ourselves up for judgement by others, which creates enormous fears of inadequacy. We then try harder and so repeat the same self-defeating behaviour.

Consequences of perfectionism

Being a perfectionist has a negative effect on many aspects of our lives, says Richard Zwolinski, a counsellor and author of *Therapy Revolution*. Here are some of the ways this behaviour can create damage to ourselves and our lives:

- *Depression* The constant struggle for perfection combined with the inevitable failure to meet that goal can lead to feelings of depression. Studies have found perfectionism to be related to increased depression, suicidal ideas, loss of self-control, shame and low self-esteem.
- *Anxiety* The consequence of feeling that perfection is just out of reach is often anxiety. Striving for perfection creates a fear of failure, and when the results are less than perfect we feel the only way to relieve those anxious feelings is to try harder, do more, be better, which in turn creates more anxiety.
- *Compulsive behaviour* The inability to tolerate imperfection can cause some people to develop obsessive or compulsive behaviours in which there's a constant drive to escape the uncomfortable feeling of being imperfect. These behaviours can include excessive hand washing or grooming, or even repeated plastic surgeries.
- *Poor relationships* Our need for approval and acceptance blinds us to the needs and wishes of others. Demanding perfection and

criticizing others creates problems. All too often we sabotage ourselves because we end up pushing others away when it's their love we so desperately want.

- *Disappointment* No one is perfect. Perfection is an unattainable goal, and striving for it inevitably leads to disappointment and negative feelings about ourselves. We're living constantly in a state of depression, anxiety, frustration and feelings of low self-worth.

Perfectionist behaviour is driven by the need to be accepted. What we often overlook is that it isn't a lack of acceptance by others that creates low self-esteem, but our sense of feeling powerless to gain acceptance of ourselves.

Dimensions of perfectionism

Perfectionism should not be confused with excellence, says Miriam Adderholdt-Elliott, author of *Perfectionism*. The pursuit of excellence is a healthy enjoyment of what you're doing, feeling good about what you've learned and developing confidence as a result. People who pursue excellence bounce back from failure and disappointment quickly and with energy, keep normal anxiety and fear of failure and disapproval within bounds and use them to create energy. They see mistakes as opportunities for growth and learning and react positively to helpful criticism.

Those who pursue perfection don't enjoy the process because they're afraid of failing and criticize themselves no matter how well they do. They see mistakes as evidence of their unworthiness and consequently become overly defensive when criticized.

The psychologist Randy Frost has researched perfectionism for many years and discovered that there are several facets to perfectionism:

- *Concern over mistakes* Perfectionists believe that a mistake is a failure and that others will look down on them if they make a mistake.
- *High personal standards* Perfectionists set very high standards for themselves and judge themselves according to those standards.

- *Parental expectations* Perfectionists believe that their parents have set high standards for them and aim to meet them.
- *Parental criticism* Perfectionists believe that their parents were overly critical.
- *Doubting* Perfectionists doubt their ability to accomplish their goals.
- *Organization* Perfectionists focus on order and neatness.

One of Frost's studies showed how the fear of criticism prevents perfectionists from improving. Students were asked to reword a passage from an introductory composition text without changing its meaning or deleting any important ideas. The results showed that those participants who were high in perfectionism scored lower on the writing test. This may be because perfectionists seem to be motivated by fear of failure and new tasks are seen as opportunities for failure. This negative belief tends to create the poor results perfectionists fear the most.

The researchers and psychologists Paul Hewitt and Gordon Flett developed another definition of perfectionism encompassing three different types:

1 *Self-orientated perfectionists* This type adheres to standards while striving for perfection and is highly motivated to avoid failure, the result of which brings intense self-evaluation.
2 *Other-orientated perfectionists* These perfectionists set unrealistic standards for others, including family, friends and co-workers, and maintain strict evaluations of their performances.
3 *Socially prescribed perfectionists* This type believes that others hold unrealistic expectations for them they can never live up to. They feel external pressure to be perfect to be valued, and believe others evaluate them critically.

   Socially prescribed perfectionism combines both pressure and a sense of helplessness and hopelessness, explains Flett. People in this category tend to feel that the better they do, the better they're expected to do.

Hewitt and Flett developed the Perfectionistic Self-Presentation Scale (PSPS) to measure how perfectionists deal with their perfectionistic drives. They found three ways perfectionists try to cope:

1 By displaying themselves as perfectionists. This includes striving to look and behave in a perfect manner in an attempt to appear capable, moral, competent and successful to others. The goal is to gain a positive reputation, respect and admiration.

2 By avoiding situations in which they might appear imperfect. This behaviour is based on the desire to avoid displaying any imperfections and includes efforts to prevent others from seeing any shortcomings, mistakes, inabilities or failures and covering up any flaws. In this way they believe they'll avoid others' disapproval.

3 By not discussing situations in which they've been imperfect. This third perfectionistic style is also avoidant and suggests they are unlikely to express concerns or admit mistakes to others through fear of rejection. This type can be less expressive generally in social situations through fear of being negatively judged or criticized.

Unfortunately none of our perfectionistic attempts to improve our self esteem works because healthy self-esteem doesn't come through achievement or external validation. Research suggests that people with low self-esteem usually try to boost their feelings of self-worth through public interaction with others, whereas people with high self-esteem manage their feelings about themselves within themselves; that is, through self-acceptance rather than the acceptance of others. Depending on others' judgement of you will necessarily create feelings of anxiety, depression, frustration, inadequacy and lower your self-esteem even further. Positive self-esteem can only develop when you believe you're a good, capable, loveable person no matter how successful or perfect you are.

The mindful way – non-judgement

Mindfulness teaches us to look at all things objectively, without judgement. In this way we accept things as they are without needing to improve or change them. Releasing judgement doesn't mean you approve of things that violate your values. It simply accepts things. Bhante Gunaratana, the author of *Mindfulness in Plain English*, explains that 'Mindfulness is objective, but not cold or unfeeling. It's the wakeful experience of life, an alert participation in the ongoing process of living.'

Most of us judge our experiences as either good or bad. The meeting at work was good; the drive home was bad. The kids are being good; the news on TV is bad. These judgements are often inaccurate interpretations of what is happening around us and yet quickly influence our thoughts and feelings. We feel bad about ourselves and the way we respond to people and to situations, and we judge ourselves and others for those responses.

The psychiatrist Rebecca Gladding suggests that we should not judge ourselves for the thoughts that arise in our minds because we can't control which thoughts or desires appear. They appear out of our subconscious mind and without our awareness. It's when we bring our awareness to the thoughts we're having that we can then choose how to respond to them. The key is not to suppress, deny or avoid our thoughts but to accept them without judging ourselves for them. Our behaviour then becomes a mindful, aware action instead of a reaction to our fears.

If we have perfectionistic behaviours we can often feel anxious and insecure because we're allowing other people to judge us and because we're judging ourselves. The struggle to be perfect demands that our self-esteem is based on other people's view of us and our perception of whether that view is good or bad; whether it's good enough. When we approach our lives non-judgementally we're no longer subjecting ourselves to scrutiny, waiting for the verdict to determine whether or not we're worthy of love and acceptance. We can simply accept ourselves, our experiences, our failures and successes and other people just as they are, neither good nor bad, without pride or shame. And that acceptance is what dissolves the anxiety, the fear and the need to keep trying to win approval. Accepting yourself without judgement means you already have that approval. You're already enough, just as you are. As the Zen priest Dogen Zenji said, 'To be in harmony with the wholeness of things is to not have anxiety over our imperfections.'

When Susan's mother came for dinner, Susan took a deep breath before showing her into the sitting room. For a moment she worried what her mother would think about their furniture and their decorating and what she'd made for dinner – her thoughts began to make her feel anxious.

Taking another deep breath, she became aware she was worrying about her mother's judgements of her and the judgements she was making about herself. She knew she wanted the dinner to be perfect so her mother would think well of her.

Realizing these thoughts were making her nervous she decided to let them go. Her mother did criticize the way she'd cooked the potatoes and said she didn't like her new hairstyle, but Susan accepted her comments as her mother's, not as a judgement about her own worth. She knew she was a good, kind, hard-working person. She knew the dinner wasn't perfect but she decided to enjoy the meal with her family anyway, without blaming herself for her mistakes. When the meal was over she realized she felt more relaxed and happy than she would have if she'd been criticizing herself all evening for not being perfect.

Non-judgemental exercises

Mindfulness practices such as meditation can help bring your thoughts into the present moment and calm your thinking so you're focused only on the experience rather than worrying about whether it's good or bad and whether you'll be judged as a result.

By focusing on the moment you can also learn to stop thinking about the mistakes you've made in the past and feeling anxious about the approval or rejection you may receive from others in the future. That worry is what erodes self-esteem. Letting go of the past and the future and focusing on the present in a non-judgemental way can help us see that there's only now. The belief that we're not good enough is just a thought we've created, which in turn creates feelings of anxiety and fear, driving us to more thoughts of our inadequacy and more fear in a self-perpetuating cycle.

Breathe

Like meditation, focusing on our breathing helps to keep us grounded in the present moment. It lowers your heart rate and calms you down, allowing you to relax and think more clearly and slowly. When you're focused on your breathing you're letting go of the judgements about the past and worries about the future and simply accepting yourself as you are now. You can practise a simple breathing exercise several times during the day as well as any time you're feeling anxious. Anxiety over being perfect can easily lead to our feeling panic and wanting to do something to alleviate those feelings, which usually causes us to engage in more perfectionistic thoughts and behaviours. Breathing gives you a chance to stop that cycle, slow down your thoughts and refocus your energy and your thoughts on accepting yourself without judgement.

Notice

Mindfulness encourages us to pay attention to the anxious thoughts and judgements we bring to our experiences. Judgements are just thoughts, and thoughts conjure up feelings. When we assign judgement to ourselves or to our experiences we're allowing our feelings to flood those experiences. When we judge ourselves we're bringing feelings to our sense of self-worth, and usually those feelings are negative, critical and damaging. Most of our thoughts happen automatically, so bringing an awareness to them allows us to notice when we're judging ourselves and others and to bring our focus gently back to the present and to acceptance of all things, just as they are.

Listen

We're often unaware of what we're thinking and how judgemental we are towards ourselves and others. By listening to the words you say, you'll find a window to the beliefs of your subconscious mind; in other words, you'll hear yourself say what you truly believe. Listen to yourself speak and see if you can hear yourself using words like 'right' and 'wrong', 'fair', 'stupid', 'lazy', 'perfect', 'bad' or 'terrible', says Christy Matta, a mindfulness trainer. These are judgement words. If you can catch yourself saying them you can become aware that you're judging yourself and others harshly. The next time you hear yourself use these kinds of words, tell yourself you're not good or bad or lazy or stupid. Focus instead on how you feel. Do you feel hurt, afraid or angry? Accept any feelings you may have. It's all right to feel them and you're all right just as you are.

Listening without judgement also involves listening to others so that we hear the intended message rather than our own interpretation of what's being said. If our self-esteem is low we tend to interpret almost everything everyone says as an attack because we feel we must have failed in some way. We then turn on whoever is speaking and lash out, often blaming them and criticizing them as a way of avoiding facing our flaws or mistakes.

The key, says Nathan Cobb, a counsellor, is to listen and try to understand what the other person is feeling and what he or she needs. For example, if your partner tells you he or she was hurt by something you said, it doesn't mean you're a bad person. It means your partner is upset by something. It isn't about whether you're a bad wife or husband or a failure, it's just the way your partner feels because of his or her own experiences. The more you can let go of your judgements about what your partner is saying and your assumptions that you're being judged, the easier it will be to give your partner what he or she needs and to gain the self-acceptance you need.

Letting go of judgement mindfully

Elisha Goldstein, a mindfulness author, suggests that when we or others around us feel understood and cared about, we all gain a sense of acceptance. He offers the following four steps to help let go of judgement when we interact with others:

1 *Put judgement aside* Be aware that you're instantly judging others as soon as you see them. We evaluate their skin colour, their style, the expression on their face and often interpret them negatively. Let your judgements go for a moment.
2 *See the person* Whatever you may believe about others or what they may be thinking about you, try to see them as just other people, like you, with their own fears, failures, dreams, hopes and desires.
3 *Ask yourself what they want* What does everyone want? To be treated kindly, compassionately, fairly and with a sense of acceptance and belonging.
4 *Act* When you let go of judgement you can choose to act instead of react. Knowing we all want acceptance means you can smile at others, listen to them, offer to help and show you care.

When we listen without judgement we let go of our interpretations of how others are judging us and recognize that what others say is about them, not about us. When we hear feedback or criticism from others we often feel they're judging not just our actions but who we are, which means our self-esteem is always at stake. Non-judgement allows us to surrender the demands we make on others as well as on ourselves, so we don't have to try to be perfect or worry about what others may think. We can just accept others as they are. And we can accept ourselves.

6

Criticism or compassion

Compassion doesn't mean you allow others to ignore your needs and feelings and put others' needs before your own. It means you're setting the standard for open, honest communication at a level where everyone's feelings and needs matter.

'I don't think these cupboards are hung properly,' said Susan to Tom one Saturday afternoon. 'You haven't done it right.'

He'd just spent the day putting the new cupboards in the kitchen.

'What do you mean?' he said. 'They're fine.'

'Look at this,' said Susan, opening and closing a door. 'It's not closing properly.'

'Of course it is,' said Tom, taking hold of the door. 'You're just not doing it right.'

What is sensitivity to criticism?

People with low self-esteem are often very sensitive to criticism. We assume others see us negatively because we see ourselves negatively. We all tend to believe others think about us the same way we think about ourselves. This is true whatever our level of self esteem. So people who think of themselves as intelligent, kind and caring generally believe others think of them that way. Likewise those who believe themselves weak, stupid, incompetent or unlovable assume others see them the same way.

Low self-esteem can cause people to respond negatively to criticism because they feel they have no choice but to defend themselves – they hear every comment as an attack. The problem is not that they're inherently inadequate or unworthy but that they *believe* they are and assume others feel the same way. Consequently they're often quick to defend themselves, criticize themselves for their flaws and mistakes or lash out and criticize others – all of which lower their self-esteem even further.

A recent study published in *USA Today* mentioned PsychTests, an online provider of psychological assessments, and used their Sensitivity to Criticism Test to show that those who tend to be defensive about criticism are less happy with their job, have low performance ratings and low self-esteem. It also found that women are more likely to take criticism personally and be hard on themselves for not doing something well. Men were more likely to convince themselves that the critic is wrong and argue with the critique. In some cases people will spend a lot of time and energy building a case against the critic and in their own defence. For both men and women, however, said the researchers, those with low self-esteem tend to ignore the constructive feedback of the critique and focus on the criticism.

Why do we criticize others?

Feeling a lack of control is one of the hallmarks of low self-esteem. Unfortunately, the tactics used to regain control, such as criticizing, only make things worse. In an attempt to feel better about themselves and feel more in control, some people will criticize others, putting others down to build themselves up. Over time this creates a self-defeating cycle of unsociable behaviour and deteriorating feelings of self-worth.

According to the marriage and family therapist Neil Rosenthal, people with low self-esteem often try to erect a barrier around themselves – an attempt to prevent others finding out how inadequate or shamed they really feel and protect themselves from criticisms and judgements. They're afraid others will find out how unacceptable they are, even if it's not true. When they're criticized it can feel as though someone is breaking through this barrier and seeing all the flaws behind the perfect façade. People with low self-esteem will naturally feel exposed and defenceless and often react to this 'invasion' with defence tactics, anger, withdrawal or aggressive, critical attacks.

Where does sensitivity to criticism come from?

This behaviour, explains Neil Rosenthal, begins in childhood. Children continually made to feel inadequate or inferior in some way will learn to erect a wall around themselves as protection against hurtful attacks. This tactic usually works – for a while – because any further criticism is met with anger, blame or defensive tactics.

However, by adulthood they have become so sensitive to any criticism that they tend to go on the attack and criticize others, whether they're being criticized or not. Those with low self-esteem believe they're always going to be criticized and so react critically as a defence, even when someone tries to help. They only *hear* criticism, not a request or a concern, and respond with criticism, withdrawal, anger or blame. If both partners in a relationship have low self-esteem, the cycle of criticism and withdrawal or anger can become the focus of the relationship.

How does our reaction to criticism affect us?

This kind of reactive behaviour not only tends to reinforce our negative beliefs about ourselves – such as the belief that we're not good enough – but also prevents us getting close to others. It prevents others sharing their feelings, needs and concerns with us and prevents us communicating in a loving, effective way. Over time, any sense of intimacy and connection will be lost – we grow apart.

What's important to remember is that constructive criticism isn't about who you are as a person, but about what you're doing. Criticism can be very advantageous because it helps you to learn and see where you've made mistakes. One of the best ways to learn something, for anyone, is by making mistakes. According to Elly Prior, a counsellor, you can't learn something new without making mistakes, because old ways of doing things are imbedded in our brain, which has to create new neural pathways for the messages about a new skill or behaviour to flow through. What that means is that learning new things is not easy – it takes practice, and we will all make mistakes along the way. But however many mistakes you make, you still deserve to be loved, appreciated and respected. The most important person to believe that is you.

The mindful way – compassion

When we feel criticized and automatically react with anger or criticism we're ignoring the needs and feelings of others. One of the worst aspects of low self-esteem is the damage it does to the people we care about. We're desperately trying to get them to think well of us, to care about us, love us and appreciate us, and yet all too often we treat them with disrespect, insensitivity and harm.

But when we allow ourselves a moment to breathe, relax and think about how we want to respond, we can choose the path of compassion, with the understanding that everyone has needs and feelings and we all need to be treated gently – including ourselves. Practising mindfulness can help us become more compassionate, in part because it encourages us to slow down, which dissolves the stress and busyness that make us blind to others' needs.

Compassion doesn't mean you allow others to ignore your needs and feelings and put others' needs before your own. It means you're setting the standard for open, honest communication at a level where *everyone's* feelings and needs matter.

The biological basis of compassion

While it's not yet entirely clear how it works, recent studies have suggested that mindful meditation may create changes in the brain that can boost our compassion for others. In a study published in the journal *Mindfulness*, a group was assigned nine 75-minute mindfulness meditation sessions over eight weeks. At the end of the training the meditation group showed improvements in their empathy and compassion and a reduction in stress levels.

Several studies have shown that compassion seems to be an innate trait in humans. One published in the journal *Psychological Science* showed that training adults in compassion meditation makes them significantly more altruistic towards others. In this meditation, participants focused on compassionate thoughts and feelings towards a loved one, themselves and someone with whom they'd had difficulty. The study is the first to link behavioural changes with measurable changes in the brain, shedding light on why compassionate thoughts lead to compassionate deeds. When we focus on helping someone else, said the researchers, the brain's reward system is activated – in other words, showing compassion for others naturally makes us feel good. When we focus on our own negative emotions and defensive behaviour, we become less focused on others' needs and less compassionate.

Further studies have shown that when we feel compassion for others, our heart rate goes down, allowing us to curb the urge to fight or flee and instead turn towards others and try to soothe them. Compassion also seems to trigger the release of oxytocin, a chemical in our bodies that increases our feelings of warmth and connection to others. Oxytocin is released through breastfeeding, hand holding and massage, but compassion can activate it as well. Compassion can therefore create a positive cycle in which a kind word or gesture releases positive feelings, and those positive feelings motivate us to be more compassionate.

Can we learn compassion?

While compassion might be built into our brains, it's also something that can be developed with practice, just like exercise or learning to play an instrument. Parents who encourage their children to think about the consequences of their actions and how their actions have harmed others, as well as set a good example of compassion, tend to raise children who are more likely to help others.

However, it can be difficult to feel compassion for other people when we haven't had this positive experience ourselves, especially if it was absent during our formative years. Some people have experienced nothing but criticism and as a result have never really felt safe. Consequently any expressions of kindness and compassion sound so strange and threatening that they find it difficult to trust.

In a study in the journal *Clinical Psychology and Psychotherapy*, researchers found that compassionate mind training significantly helped people with high levels of self-criticism and feelings of shame. Results showed significant reductions in depression, anxiety, self-criticism, shame, inferiority and submissive behaviour.

There were also increases in participants' ability to soothe themselves and focus on feelings of warmth and reassurance for themselves.

Even if we did not grow up with positive examples or expressions of compassion, our minds were made to give and receive compassion. It's something we can all learn with practice.

According to the psychotherapist B. Raven Lee, in peak meditative states there's a reduction in activity level in the orientation association area of the brain. Researchers have suggested that this results in a decrease in the boundary between our self and others, which may account, says Lee, in meditators feeling a sense of oneness and compassion with all living beings.

Mindfulness offers a choice

When someone offers you a criticism or points out the mistakes you made, you have the option of responding in one of two ways:

- either you can react because you feel threatened and attacked;
- or you can take a moment to pause, breathe and reflect.

Reacting to criticism will leave both people feeling more upset. In addition, your self-esteem will take another hit because you're defending your negative belief about yourself. If someone tells you your presentation was stupid, reacting to that only confirms your belief that you feel you're stupid. Mindfulness reminds us we have a choice in how we respond. This is key to building your self-esteem because it enables you to feel in control of yourself and your life, rather than fearful, defenceless and out of control.

This choice only becomes apparent when you stop for a moment and breathe. Just breathe in and then breathe out. Keep focusing on your breathing until you feel calm. According to the relationship expert John Gottman, it usually takes about 20 minutes for our heart rate to come down to normal when we're upset or stressed. During this time it's best to avoid discussing the problem any further until you're feeling calm.

When we get upset or hurt or angry by criticism our emotions get in the way of our thinking and we tend to react in self-defeating ways that are intended to protect us but result in a greater sense of fear. But by taking a moment to breathe we can act mindfully, with our full consciousness and awareness, which then allows us to choose how we want to proceed.

Once you're calm you can then choose whether to accept the criticism or not. Simply breathe and then ask yourself these questions:

- Is this person actually attacking who I am?
- Or are they showing me where I went wrong? Are they offering a suggestion that will help me improve in some way?

Some critiques are useful, pointing out areas for potential growth you may not have seen yourself. Others may not be helpful. The key is to recognize that the choice is yours. Whatever someone is offering belongs to them, and it's up to you to decide whether you want to accept it or not. Whether you choose to ignore it or to take it, your self-esteem is given a boost because you're in control and making the choice yourself. Your self-esteem is not in jeopardy because it's not personal.

Conversely, when you react your self-esteem is at risk because you're assuming the criticism is an attack on your character. Even if someone *is* attacking your character, you're the only person who can judge whether you're good, acceptable, adequate or loveable. So that means anything others say is about them and their views – it's not about you. But you can choose to learn from it.

For example, if someone tells you you're lazy, fat, ugly, a terrible accountant or a bad parent, you don't have to react. You have a choice. If you have low self-esteem you'll tend to get upset by these kinds of comments, not because they're actually true but because you believe them to be true. But remember they're a reflection of the other person, who is probably saying them because that's how they feel about themselves. So you can choose whether to accept them or not. Are they going to help you improve or learn in some way? The answer to most such unfair criticism is no – they're only going to make you feel bad. You can choose not to accept them. It's not always easy to ignore such hurtful remarks – especially when they come from someone you care about – but they have nothing to do with you or your worth as a person. Only you can decide that. When you have compassion for yourself it's easier to recognize that negative remarks aren't true. When you have compassion for others you can recognize that the person criticizing you is probably hurting too and there's no need to go on the attack yourself.

Compassion at work

Constructive criticism is meant to help you, guide you and develop your strengths. If someone tells you your presentation at work was disorganized and that others found it hard to follow, again you have a choice. You can get defensive or criticize that person or you can take a deep breath and ask yourself whether it would be helpful to consider these remarks. With a compassionate perspective you can recognize that this person is only trying to help you. Perhaps you've never given a presentation before and you were nervous, but you'd like to do better. So accepting this criticism might be helpful. You might ask for help with making your presentation more organized. It can also be helpful to ask for criticism when you're trying to learn something new.

If you can remember that constructive criticism is not a statement about your worth as a person but simply about your presentation, you can gain the knowledge and skills you need to improve. Using information to improve your skills will lead to a better performance next time, and that will lead to greater positive feelings about your skills, your ability to learn and cope, and to better feelings about yourself.

Whether you're asking for feedback or are faced with criticism, you need to feel calm enough to make a choice as to whether you want to accept it or not. You also need time to think about it. Mindfulness is about slowing things down and not rushing – you can only make decisions when you've considered all things consciously. Be sure to take a deep breath and remember it's not a personal attack. Give yourself time to think about what you want to do next based on the information you've received.

Compassion in relationships

Many people feel threatened and become defensive when they think others don't understand them or have little interest in taking their point of view seriously. Listening, expressing understanding of your partner's concerns and offering your confirmation that those concerns are valid is a way of responding with compassion. Likewise, instead of reacting to what you perceive as criticism, ask for more information from your partner – ask questions and try to clarify any misunderstandings.

For example, if your partner tells you you drive too fast, instead of reacting negatively to this criticism by defending yourself and criticizing the way he does the dishes, you could respond with compassion. Ask why it bothers him. He could respond that he worries about your safety, in which case you might decide it would be a good idea to slow down. Likewise, you could tell your partner you felt criticized by his remarks and so perhaps that's why you responded by criticizing the way he does the dishes. He might just appreciate your honesty and openness and feel inspired to move closer to you rather than retreat or put up barriers.

> 'That curtain rail in the bedroom isn't straight,' Susan told Tom the following weekend.
>
> 'Really?' He stood back and looked at it. 'It looks straight to me.'
>
> 'Can you see how the right side is higher than the left? Just a few inches.'
>
> 'Oh, you're right. I hadn't noticed. Wait, let me get my cordless drill and I'll fix it.'
>
> 'It's not a big deal. It's just that my mother's coming next week and I want it to be just right.'
>
> 'That's okay. I want it to be just right too. After all, we live here! What do you think now?'
>
> 'That's it! You've done it! Thank you. You've done a great job with this room.'
>
> 'I'm not the greatest handyman in the world,' Tom laughed, 'but I try my best.'
>
> Susan kissed him. 'It looks beautiful.'

'We all want to be loved,' says the clinical psychologist Lisa Firestone in the article '8 Ways to Tell if You're a *Truly* Compassionate Person', published on <huffingtonpost.com> and written by Lindsay Holmes, 'but what actually feels good to us is feeling loving,' and that means being compassionate towards others. In one study researchers found that our sense of compassion increases when there's a common connection with another person. According to the psychologist David DeSteno: 'If we can draw an association between someone else and ourselves, the compassion we feel for his or her suffering is amplified greatly.'

Once you can understand each other's real concerns, needs and feelings, you can choose to act less critically and defensively and more compassionately by showing respect for each other during moments of tension. In this way both partners feel heard, validated, understood, accepted and loved. When we create a communication strategy that allows everyone to feel *safe*, we can free ourselves to feel and offer compassion to those we care about. The more compassionate we feel towards others, the better we feel about ourselves.

In the words of the Buddhist monk Thich Nhat Hanh:

> When we are peaceful and happy, we will not create suffering in others. When we work to alleviate the suffering in others, we feel peaceful and happy. Practice is not just for ourselves, but for others and the whole of society.

7

People-pleasing or connecting

To be beautiful means to be yourself. You don't need to be accepted by others. You need to accept yourself.

Thich Nhat Hanh

Susan was exhausted, but when a woman from her office asked her to be a volunteer for a fundraiser that weekend, she happily agreed. She'd also agreed to walk her neighbour's dog while he was on holiday and to take care of her best friend's children one night a week. It made her feel good when people asked her for help. She felt people needed her. She liked thinking of herself as the happy, cheerful friend everyone could always count on. Besides, she wanted people to like her and she'd been raised to believe it was selfish to put yourself first. Sometimes she thought about coming up with an excuse to avoid another commitment, but she felt so uneasy and anxious about it, she always gave in. The only trouble was that now she was so tired and had no time to herself, she was beginning to feel resentful, which made her think badly of herself.

What is people-pleasing?

While low self-esteem can often lead us to become angry and attack others, it can also make us hard on ourselves. For some people, their efforts to feel good about who they are cause them to try to make others like them, at any cost. If they're rejected or hurt they believe it's because they aren't nice enough. Appearing friendly, caring, courteous, helpful and supportive, a tendency towards people-pleasing may seem nice, but it's usually nice taken too far, to the extent that people-pleasers completely neglect their own needs.

In her book *The Disease to Please*, Harriet Braiker provides a list of self-destructive thoughts and beliefs most people-pleasers adopt – what she calls the 'Ten Commandments of People-Pleasing':

1 I should always do what others want, expect or need from me.
2 I should take care of everyone around me whether they ask for help or not.
3 I should always listen to everyone's problems and try my best to solve them.
4 I should always be nice and never hurt anyone's feelings.
5 I should always put other people first, before me.
6 I should never say 'no' to anyone who needs or requests something of me.
7 I should never disappoint anyone or let others down in any way.
8 I should always be happy and upbeat and never show any negative feelings to others.
9 I should always try to please other people and make them happy.
10 I should try never to burden others with my own needs or problems.

While this kind of behaviour makes other people happy, it fails to fill the void people-pleasers feel inside themselves. People-pleasing behaviours are a mask for the pain and negative beliefs people-pleasers really feel, says the psychologist Leon Seltzer. Beneath their cheerful persona they're terrified of rejection, and fear losing others' approval, feeling lonely and isolated, undeserving, inferior and inadequate. Believing that giving other people what they want will earn them the love and respect they long for, they become incapable of feeling good about themselves without the validation of others.

People-pleasers have spent so much time deferring to other people's needs and demands that they often no longer know their own but end up feeling frustrated, used, inadequate and angry because their needs continue to be ignored. By continually putting others' needs before their own, people-pleasers put others in a position of authority over them. They expect that by being nice to people they'll earn their acceptance and protect themselves from being hurt.

This is why people-pleasing is not only a symptom of low self-esteem but a cause. We become increasingly anxious about getting the approval of others, while allowing them to take us for granted. In this way, says Seltzer, people-pleasing is like an addiction – the need for approval becomes insatiable, while never leading to the love we seek.

Over time other people can become more demanding, taking more of what they can get and leaving you exhausted, drained and neglected. The need to please others also makes people-pleasers the target of bullies, narcissists and controlling types. Subconsciously, people-pleasers are often attracted to controlling people because they'll make all the decisions and take control, which is what they feel most comfortable with. But the more they give to others and ignore themselves, the more inadequate, victimized and helpless they feel, and the more they struggle to meet the ever-increasing demands of others, lowering their self-esteem even further.

Denying your own needs and repressing your thoughts and feelings for a long time can lead to resentment and anger, but many feel they can't express themselves out of fear of rejection or condemnation by others. Failing to be assertive in any situation, unable to make decisions independently and seeking only to avoid conflict, many people-pleasers lose touch with who they are and what they want.

For some people this results in passive-aggressive behaviour – anger expressed through subtle negative actions, such as being chronically late, agreeing to do something but not making an effort or through biting comments and sarcasm. While this anger and resentment is understandable, passive-aggression only works to upset other people and destroy relationships, ultimately pushing away the people you want to get close to.

Why do we become people-pleasers?

People-pleasers generally felt loved as children only when they were conforming to the needs and wishes of their parents, says Seltzer. They may have been praised only when they performed well in school or in sports. Perhaps they were criticized for who they were – for example, their parents may have wanted them to be more sociable when in fact the child in question was an introvert.

Parents can also be overprotective and answer for children, with the result that they never learn to express their own opinions and become dependent on others to do so for them.

Ignoring their parents' wishes or expressing their own needs was usually met with criticism or withdrawal of attention, caring or understanding, leaving the child to feel not only disapproved of but rejected and abandoned.

Children in this situation quickly learn that sacrificing their own needs, feelings and desires – that is, their own sense of self – was the price to pay for love and acceptance. To assert their own individualism was met not only with disdain and disapproval but triggered feelings of shame, guilt and humiliation. But continually sacrificing their own needs for the needs and desires of others led to deep-rooted feelings of unworthiness and low self-esteem.

Most people with low self-esteem came from families with poor boundaries, says Marilyn Sorensen, the author of *Breaking the Chain of Low Self-Esteem*. Boundaries are limits we set to protect ourselves and to let others know what is or isn't acceptable for us. Growing up, people-pleasers may not have learned how to develop healthy boundaries because their individuality or creativity was discouraged or their personal space and possessions were violated. They may not have been allowed to express their opinions, preferences or make choices. Consequently they grew up not knowing what their opinions are, feeling afraid to express themselves and confused about what is acceptable behaviour.

The psychologist Jay Earley suggests that our environment and culture also puts pressure on people to conform to the wishes of others, encouraging us – particularly women – to put other people first and teaching us that our own feelings and needs don't count.

It's only when we begin to put our needs and feelings in greater priority that we can begin to move past the people-pleasing behaviours that keep us tied to others' approval. And it's only when we recognize that the love, acceptance and respect we're so longing for can only come from within ourselves that we can see our self-esteem grow. What we need to recognize, says Harriet Braiker, is that each of us is the only person whose acceptance we really need.

Taking the steps to put yourself first and give yourself the love you need requires assertiveness, which means taking action, setting limits, asking for what you want and reaching out for connection with – rather than subservience to – others. But when a certain kind of behaviour has become a pattern over time it can be very difficult to change. When that behaviour was helpful to us growing up, it can be even harder to change, even when we want to, because on some subconscious level we feel it has worked for us.

It's important to expect feelings of hesitancy, nervousness, guilt and ambivalence when trying to change a behavioural pattern, says Leon Seltzer. The reason many people don't change is that these uncomfortable feelings arise whenever they try to act in a self-affirming way, and they assume their feelings are telling them they're doing something wrong. They're actually telling you that you need to act in a way that's more connected with who you are, rather than with someone else.

Fortunately, awareness of our thoughts and feelings and assertive connection to ourselves is what mindfulness can bring to your relationships and your life.

The mindful way – connected

Mindfulness is the practice of paying attention to what is happening around you and within you and about being connected to your experiences and to yourself. Since long-term people-pleasing involves doing what others want so they'll love you, you can't be accepted or loved for who you are. Who you are has become what everyone else wants. In this way you eventually become disconnected from your inner life and from yourself.

Connected to the real you

When you're connected to yourself you realize you have everything you need within you, including the love, peace, respect and acceptance you've been searching for. You no longer need to look outside yourself for approval; you already know you're all right. Once you become aware of yourself and love yourself for who you are, you're then in a place of happiness from which you can joyfully connect to others in a loving, harmonious way.

Connection to others

Many of us feel alone and disconnected from others and the love and joy that seem so abundant in life yet always somehow out of our reach. When we have low self-esteem we struggle to make others like us and approve of us, and we try to make ourselves good enough to be worthy of love and attention and connection. Yet we find ourselves struggling even harder.

Studies show that people who feel more connected to others have higher self-esteem and lower rates of anxiety and depression. They're also more empathic, more trusting and co-operative and, consequently, others are more open to trusting and co-operating with them.

However, research reveals that the psychological and physical benefits of social connection come not from the number of friends we have but our *sense of connection* towards others. What this means is that connection comes from within us and our ability to share our true selves with others.

Mindfulness exercises to build connection

According to Micki Fine, the author of *The Need to Please*, mindfulness can help you develop a sense of connection and reduce your people-pleasing ways by allowing you to stop the autopilot thinking and behaviour that keeps you jumping to please others without thinking of your own needs.

Breathe

If someone asks you to help at the local school, you might normally say yes without question. By practising mindfulness you can learn to pause, take a deep breath and let go of the fear that causes you to seek others' approval. When you take time to breathe you become aware that you have a choice to react out of fear or to act according to your own needs.

Develop awareness

By developing your awareness of your thoughts you can recognize your fear talking to you, telling you things like 'I'd better agree or she won't like me' or 'It's not very nice to say no'. By bringing non-judgemental attention to the present moment you can notice the feelings that arise in your body and the anxiety you may be feeling. Giving in to other people's demands is simply a way of soothing that anxiety, but it keeps you a prisoner of your own fear.

Instead of trying to soothe the anxiety, recognize it as a sign that you're feeling forced to do something you don't want to do. Awareness allows you to recognize that the fear-based feelings that arise come from the child within you. As an adult you can choose how you want to respond and decide to put your own needs first. You can choose to see yourself in a loving way. Seltzer suggests gently reassuring the inner child that it's all right to assert your needs and desires and say no when it feels like the right thing – these needs and desires are important and it's all right to express them, even when they differ from someone else's.

Reconnect with your body

You can reconnect with your body through the practice of mindful walking or mindful yoga, says Micki Fine. Feeling connected to your body is critical to loving yourself since the body is where you feel anxiety and fear and where you feel love. The more connected you are to your body the more you'll be in touch with what you really want and what you really need.

Meditate

Taking a few moments every day simply to be still and focus on your breathing is an excellent way to help you stay connected and let go of the struggle for acceptance. The aim of meditation is not to enable you to become a master meditator or even to have a life-changing experience but to develop an awareness that you have everything you need inside you and that you're all right. When you can treat yourself with the same respect and kindness and compassion you show to others, you'll feel calmer, safer and more secure with yourself.

The loving-kindness meditation from Chapter 1 encourages a sense of gentle acceptance of yourself. Set aside 20 minutes for this meditation; whatever feelings or thoughts arise, respond to them with kindness.

Susan decided to sign up for a yoga class. It was the first thing she'd ever really done just for herself. She felt guilty at first and worried about the time she was taking away from others. But as she learned to breathe she slowly relaxed and began to feel more connected to the person she really was rather than just a helper, a giver, a servant to others. She noticed how peaceful she felt when she was calm. Spending time in yoga helped her to get back in touch with her own body so that she began to notice when she felt out of sorts – such as when her heart started pounding or her hands would perspire when someone asked her to do something. She'd take a deep breath and focus on the moment. She knew this anxious feeling was her own fear of being rejected, and she knew she would not reject herself. She'd love herself the way she wanted others to love her. She practised saying no when she didn't want to take on another job for someone. And she said yes to the volunteer work because it was something she believed in but had never had the courage to speak out about before.

If we connect with ourselves in a loving way, knowing we have the love inside us that we need, we'll be able to take care of others and ourselves out of love rather than fear.

8

Lack of assertiveness or participation

The act of participation in your own life is vital to the development of your self-esteem because it enables you to heal yourself of your own painful experiences.

Susan had always felt frustrated when Tom came home from work late without calling. She'd tried everything she could think of, including ignoring him when he did come home, burning the dinner, or arriving late to their appointments with their financial advisor. But nothing seemed to work. All she knew was that she was feeling increasingly frustrated, resentful and angry and something had to change. Somehow, she decided, she'd think up something to do to Tom that would really get his attention.

What is assertiveness?

Assertiveness means standing up for yourself, setting limits and acting in a way that serves your needs. It means saying no to what feels wrong to you. It means initiating action, taking risks and working towards goals. Assertiveness is expressing your opinion and speaking up for what you think is right. You need to let the people you love know what your needs are and expect that they'll take some responsibility in helping to fulfil them.

Jay Earley, a psychologist and expert on people-pleasing, says it's important to remember that assertiveness isn't aggression or condescension; it isn't controlling or judgemental. When you're assertive you're connected, so that you're open and accepting of other people's needs and opinions without sacrificing your own.

To be assertive you must know what you want, how you feel and what you need rather than allowing yourself to be influenced by others. Sometimes it takes time to know what you want or need, so it's important to think about what you want and to say no or ask for more time if you're unsure about a decision.

In response to a request for help, for example, you might say, 'I'll think about that and let you know' or 'Thanks, but I need to focus on my health right now.' Other people may not approve of your response, but you're approving of yourself and loving yourself, which is the best way to improve your self-esteem.

Lack of assertiveness

People with low self-esteem often avoid expressing their feelings, speaking up for themselves or asking for what they want and need. They also find it difficult to bounce back after a setback and often withdraw socially. Assertive behaviour, however, is essential for maintaining healthy relationships and developing a positive sense of self-regard.

When we tell the truth we're allowing ourselves to be vulnerable. When people have low self-esteem their sense of value about themselves comes not from within but from others. Expressing their concerns, needs and wants means risking that this might upset or anger others and they would consequently face criticism, admonishment or rejection, lowering their self-esteem even further. They also feel that whatever mistakes have been made were their fault.

Their strategy is to keep quiet, keeping their beliefs and opinions private and agreeing with everyone else to protect themselves. This lack of assertiveness, however, tends to crush their own sense of self. In some cases people with low self-esteem don't even know what they want when asked, because they've lost touch with their own needs and desires.

In addition, failing to assert yourself means that others often make unreasonable demands of you – you can become trapped in unhealthy relationships and find it difficult to leave or to change your behaviour.

Over time this passive response tends to build into frustration and anger, says the clinical psychologist Marilyn Sorensen, until it seeps out in sarcastic or biting remarks, rudeness, defensiveness or even violence.

What is lack of assertiveness?

Being assertive is a choice we can make when confronted with a situation or a person that affects our well-being. When we are assertive we're clear about how we feel, what we need and what we want, while remaining considerate of the needs, values and wants of others. A lack of assertiveness can include the following harmful beliefs and behaviours:

- you say yes when you really want to say no;
- you allow others to cross your boundaries and treat you badly;
- you feel unable to defend yourself or stand up to someone who's hurting or upsetting you;
- you express your thoughts and feelings in an apologetic way so that others easily disregard them;
- you're unable to receive negative feedback without blaming yourself;
- you're unable to receive compliments;
- you're unable to listen to others and accommodate their needs;
- you believe your needs, wants and wishes aren't as important as others';
- you have body language that includes lack of eye contact, looking down, biting your lip or crossing your arms.

Because assertiveness requires confidence, calmness and the ability to communicate your needs effectively, many people struggle to assert themselves without being too aggressive or too passive. Society also tends to discourage assertiveness, says Sorensen, and encourages people instead to 'go with the flow' and not cause trouble by speaking out. Saying what you think and disagreeing with others is often seen as selfish, demanding or rude.

But being assertive can help to improve your relationships by ensuring everyone's needs, desires and feelings are understood and treated equally. Asserting yourself means you treat yourself with as much compassion and respect as you treat others. And it means you feel more in control of your life and build your self-esteem by expressing yourself and allowing yourself to be who you are, even if it's not the same as everyone else.

Why do we become unassertive?

Assertiveness is not a character trait you're born with or without but a behaviour that's learned as you grow up. If your family, friends, colleagues or authority figures responded to your attempts to express your needs with hostility, ridicule or rejection, for example, you may have learned to keep your needs quiet.

Likewise, some families or communities teach their children that they should think of others before themselves, which can lead to their feeling guilty or afraid of expressing themselves. It's important, however, not to blame your parents, siblings or others you grow up with for your lack of assertiveness – they were probably following the rules they were taught. But as an adult you have a choice and you have the ability to change the behaviours and thoughts that have been unhealthy for you.

Aggressive behaviour

While lack of assertiveness keeps our beliefs and needs locked inside us and our responses to the world passive, the opposite extreme of aggressive behaviour is just as harmful.

Many people mistake aggression for assertiveness, in the belief that the more forcefully you express your needs the more likely you are to get what you want. Aggressive behaviour includes threatening or attacking others, putting them down, using a sarcastic or condescending tone, refusing to listen, blaming, speaking loudly or making racist/sexist remarks.

But aggressive behaviour only violates other people's rights, destroys relationships and ultimately weakens your self-esteem because you know they're submitting to your will out of fear, not because of your value as a person.

Passive-aggressive behaviour

According again to Sorensen, lack of assertiveness in someone with low self-esteem can also manifest into passive-aggressive behaviour, such as manipulation, chronic lateness and gossiping. Low self-esteem can often manifest as passive-aggressive behaviour because we're too afraid to show our anger, hurt or frustration to others in case they become angry and reject us.

Passive-aggression is an *indirect* form of aggression, explains the psychologist Leon Seltzer, not necessarily a *milder* form. Because getting our needs met, our voices heard and our feelings understood is essential to the survival of our selves, of who we are as individuals, the urge to achieve this persists even when we've been bullied, coerced, threatened or punished for trying to.

While we try, subconsciously or consciously, to suppress our needs so that we might win the approval of others, our true selves often assert themselves in passive-aggressive ways that reflect the frustration and anger we really feel at not being able to be ourselves. In this way we can express our grievances while believing we're maintaining the relationships we can't afford to jeopardize. The result is that we sabotage, undermine, deceive and betray those we care about. We disappoint, withhold, disengage, make up excuses, and blame others for our own mistakes and misbehaviours.

Growing up in environments in which we could not depend on our parents to meet our needs adequately means that, even as adults, we're not comfortable depending on others. Being in a relationship necessarily requires a certain amount of dependency and so passive-aggressive people bring frustrated feelings about their unmet needs into all their relationships, always searching for security and respect but continually sabotaging the relationship out of their deep-rooted belief that their needs will never be met.

Assertive behaviour

When you're assertive you express your needs and feelings in a calm, decisive manner, without apologizing and without hurting anyone. It's a way of communicating in an open, honest manner that respects the needs and rights of both yourself and others.

When you're assertive you don't need to be angry, loud, demanding or pleading to get what you want. You state your needs and desires simply and concisely. Expressing yourself directly in the present moment also prevents resentment and worry about criticism from building up. When you take responsibility for getting your needs met by expressing them, you become less driven by the need to protect yourself and more able to relax, be yourself with confidence and listen to others' needs.

Assertiveness is not about control or dominance or submitting to the will of others – it's about expression, mutual understanding and respect.

Here are some tips provided by the Better Health Channel to help you learn to be more assertive.

- *Aim for open and honest communication* Remember to respect other people when you're sharing your feelings, wants, needs, beliefs or opinions.
- *Listen actively* Try to understand the other person's point of view and don't interrupt when they're explaining it to you.
- *Agree to disagree* Remember that having a different point of view doesn't mean you're right and the other person is wrong.
- *Avoid guilt trips* Be honest and tell others how you feel or what you want, without making accusations or making them feel guilty.
- *Stay calm* Remember to breathe, look the person in the eye, keep your face relaxed and speak in a normal voice.
- *Take a problem-solving approach to conflict* Try to see the other person as your friend, not your enemy.
- *Practise assertiveness* Talk in an assertive way in front of a mirror or with a friend. Pay attention to your body language as well as to the words you say.
- *Use 'I'* Stick with statements that include 'I' in them, such as 'I think' or 'I feel'. Don't use aggressive language such as 'you always' or 'you never'.
- *Be patient* Being assertive is a skill that needs practice. Remember that you'll do better at it at some times than at others, but you can always learn from your mistakes.

Taking action to stand up for yourself and express your own needs, beliefs and feelings is an essential step towards improving your self-esteem – it's essentially telling others, and more significantly yourself, that you're important and deserve to be heard.

The next time Tom came home late from work without calling, Susan recognized her thoughts and feelings – negative thoughts about Tom and anxious, worried and angry feelings. She became aware of her heart pounding and her hands sweating as the minutes ticked by. When Tom came home he explained he'd had a meeting and was sorry he hadn't called. Previously she'd just have nodded and said nothing but be seething with anger underneath. This time she took a deep breath, exhaled, and told Tom she felt frustrated when he didn't call to say he'd be late. She worked hard all day too and always tried to make dinner for them both. She told him she felt unappreciated when he didn't call. Tom wasn't used to Susan asserting herself in this way. He was surprised at first but appreciated her calm, open approach – more than her usual passive-aggressive tactics. He'd known she was angry about something but had no idea what. Now he knew what they were dealing with. And they could work it out together.

The mindful way – participation

Mindfulness is about being aware of what's happening in the present moment. But more than that, it's about participation in what's happening. While mindfulness encourages us to become unattached to thoughts that can induce negative feelings, it also tells us to engage, to become active and assertive in creating our own lives.

According to Marsha Linehan, the creator of Dialectical Behaviour Therapy, participation is one of the three 'what' skills of mindfulness – observing, describing and participating. The more you participate in what's happening around you in the present moment, the more you are able to take control of your own life.

Noticing negative thoughts is not a passive act, says the mindfulness expert Jon Kabat-Zinn. Awareness of your thoughts and your responses to them enables you to take action. Making choices and taking action is participation in your own life. Once you see what's happening you have the insight to choose how to proceed. In this way, he says, the real meditation practice is your life.

This act of participation in your own life is vital to the development of your self-esteem because it enables you to heal yourself of your own painful experiences rather than waiting passively for someone else to come and rescue you. You can become the hero you're waiting for.

Engaging in your everyday life in a mindful way means you choose to stay present when negative thoughts come into your mind. Mindfulness allows you to stay in the moment when your fears and unpleasant emotions arise, and gives you the strength to face them instead of allowing them to overwhelm you or drive you to try to escape.

Escape is often our first response when we're feeling negative emotions such as fear. When we lack assertiveness, we can easily become overwhelmed by stressful situations or demanding people. Most of us live on autopilot; that is, instead of choosing how to respond to a situation we simply react, and that reaction is often the easiest, quickest way to find relief, whether it comes from shopping, eating, drinking or gambling. And while these escape routes provide temporary relief from our pain, they're only temporary. In fact the pain tends to get bigger, along with our fears and our self-doubts, while our self-esteem and our belief in our own ability to cope shrinks with every encounter.

Mindful participation, on the other hand, means that when stressful, difficult or painful situations arise, or negative thoughts, worries or fears, we just let them go. This is how we can take back control of our lives and become more assertive, confident and assured of our own self-worth.

Unentangled participation

The monk Ajahn Amaro called this sort of awareness 'unentangled participation'. What this means is participating in your own life without becoming tangled up by the past or the future. It's living each moment, each experience, free from the trap of negative thoughts or feelings, from worry, fear, self-criticism, judgement, frustration, yearning or the desire to escape. It allows you to accept things as they are and live in the present moment, while being aware of the past and future concerns that have kept you tangled up in a knot of unhappiness.

When you notice the negative thoughts or feelings emerge, try looking at them as if they were objects, like birds flying in the sky. You can notice them and recognize them but they're not part of who you are – you don't have to attach yourself to them or identify yourself with them. When you can let them go in this way you're choosing to become an assertive participant in your own life and releasing yourself from the bonds of entanglement.

Letting go of the thoughts in your own mind is not always easy. We all love our stories, says Amaro, particularly the ones about ourselves. We're constantly talking to ourselves about what we've done right or what we've done wrong; what we should have done better or shouldn't have done at all; what we want to do and what we're afraid will happen. With the help of meditation, however, we can learn to recognize the thinking habits that generate these kinds of thoughts and learn to let them go.

Vipassana, or insight meditation

Vipassana is the practice of continued close attention to what you're experiencing in the present moment. The purpose of meditation is not to achieve a certain state of mind but to train your mind to focus on the moment and become aware of your own thoughts, responses and sensations in your body and your mind. This awareness develops the mind to become aware of the truth. Meditation is like exercise, so it becomes easier with repeated practice and, like exercise, the goal is not to reach the finish line but to develop the mind and body.

According to the Vipassana master Sayadaw U Pandita, when insight arises and deepens through Vipassana, or insight meditation practice, particular aspects of the truth about existence tend to be revealed in a definite order. This order is known as the progress of insight. The first insight meditators experience is usually the awareness that two distinct processes are happening together: the physical and the mental. After that you begin to see that the physical causes the mental and the mental causes the physical, such as when a mental thought of fear causes us to run away. This second insight allows us to see that life is a simple series of causes and effects. The next step is to see that they happen quickly and that they're temporary and impersonal. Pandita suggests the step-by-step practice shown in the panel overleaf.

In the same way that mindful participation enables us to let go of negative thoughts and feelings, it also provides us with the awareness of the beauty that's all around us. When we're fully participating in our lives, we suddenly notice the shapes of the leaves on the trees and smell the scent of the flowers; we see the colours of a sunset and hear the music of laughter. This awareness brings joy, calmness and an assertive participation in life that nurtures our compassion for ourselves and others and in turn develops our sense of our own self-worth and our vital part in the world.

1   Sit quietly and comfortably. The important thing is to be relaxed. To achieve peace of mind your body must be at peace, so it's important to choose a position that will be comfortable for a long time.
2   Close your eyes and focus your attention on your abdomen. Breathe normally.
3   Notice what happens in your body as you breathe in and out, as your abdomen rises and falls. You can help yourself to maintain focus by thinking to yourself the words 'rising, rising' and 'falling, falling' as they happen.
4   If your mind wanders, become aware that it's wandering and gently bring your focus back to your breathing. If a sound or other distraction interrupts you, draw your attention to the distraction, notice it and give it a label, such as 'hearing'. Labelling allows us to become more clearly aware of an experience without becoming attached to it. With a label, it becomes an object that's separate from us.
5   When the sound or distraction fades, come back to noticing the rising and falling sensation. Trying to ignore the distraction or push it away will only cause you to focus on the effort of pushing and ignoring, instead of your breathing.
6   When you decide to stop, begin with the intention to open your eyes by thinking the words 'intending, intending' and then 'opening, opening'. Notice the thought of intention and feel the physical sensation of your eyes opening, your limbs moving, your body standing.
7   Throughout the day, continue to be aware of all your activities, such as picking up a spoon, opening a door, brushing your teeth, eating.

9
Distorted sense of trust or observing

When we observe our thoughts, feelings and behaviour in a compassionate, non-judgemental way, we're able to see ourselves as we truly are.

Tom couldn't shake the anxious feeling he'd developed lately, couldn't even put his finger on it. He just felt nervous, as if he had too much energy, but also exhausted. He thought at first it was work stress but then noticed he felt worse when he came home. Usually Susan came home from work before him and he liked to see her when he opened the door. But she'd started taking a cooking class on Tuesday evenings and was often home late. Usually he was the one who was late but now he wondered if she was trying to teach him a lesson. She'd been late home on Thursday night too, although she said she'd had to stop at the grocery store on her way. But he had a terrible feeling she was being unfaithful to him. He'd heard her mention a man named Steve from her cooking class. He'd asked her about him but she'd denied any involvement. He decided he would demand the truth when she got home. In the meantime, he would check her emails, just to be sure.

What is a distorted sense of trust?

Everyone has to make choices about who or what to trust every day. Some situations are clearer than others and some days our ability to make the right decision is difficult. Feeling a certain amount of uncertainty about whom to trust and when to trust is essential to our safety and allows us to make informed decisions.

When we have low self-esteem we're more often confused about whom to trust. We often feel anxious in relationships or social situations, confused, suspicious, angry or unable to make decisions; these feelings can in turn weaken our self-esteem.

In some cases we trust anyone who's nice to us or shows us the attention we've always craved, leaving us vulnerable to being taken advantage of and betrayed even further.

In their book *Safe People*, Henry Cloud and John Townsend present some characteristics of untrustworthy people. They:

- project things on to others instead of admitting their weaknesses;
- are defensive instead of open to feedback;
- apologize but don't change their behaviour;
- demand trust instead of earning it;
- lie instead of being honest;
- resist growing and changing themselves;
- are unstable over time instead of being consistent.

At the same time we often feel unable to trust people who are genuinely trustworthy, and reject offers of support and love, as well as healthy relationships. This is because we don't believe this kind of genuine affection is real. Consistent expressions of love, kindness or even compliments feel so foreign to us that we have a hard time accepting them. We've learned that expressions of love should not be trusted.

Here are some signs that we have issues with trust:

- We might feel unable to trust our romantic partner and become jealous.
- We abandon partners before they abandon us, as we're sure they will.
- We keep others at an emotional distance and never commit.
- We find ourselves unable even to enter into a romantic relationship.
- We rush quickly into a new relationship, even before getting to know a person well.
- We often let partners off the hook, even when it's undeserved, for fear of losing them.

What is trust?

Researchers define trust as a willingness to share personal information with another person. This involves being both vulnerable enough to open up about yourself and also willing to listen to the other person and respect his or her reality. When we both listen and share, trust is built.

Listening and sharing allow us to connect to other people because, according to Henry Cloud, connection is built through being understood. When we fail to listen and instead get defensive, blame or criticize, or when we keep ourselves closed up and fail to share, trust becomes increasingly difficult and our connection to others is broken.

Trust is something that has to be earned. People with low self-esteem often trust others too quickly, before getting to know them properly. Trust can only develop over time, when we behave in a consistently trustworthy manner and are able to witness others' characters over a period of time, getting to know who they are and what they stand for.

Trust is essential to healthy relationships and a healthy social life. Social support and participation in social activities positively affects our psychological well-being and our self-esteem. Without the ability to trust, our relationships become rocky and fragile, further damaging our self-esteem.

Why can't we trust?

As we were growing up we were often sent mixed messages by those closest to us. Our parents may have told us they loved us but acted critically, judgementally or ignored us. Likewise some parents act in a loving way but never tell their children they love them. Experiencing your parents' divorce or betraying or hurting each other can also leave you feeling hesitant about trusting others. Children often feel betrayed and unable to depend on those they should have been able to trust. Someone who didn't receive adequate nurturing, affection and acceptance or who was abused, violated, or mistreated as a child will often find difficulty establishing trust as an adult.

Our social experiences with others as we grow up can also influence our later relationships. Feeling socially rejected, teased, bullied, attacked or humiliated during our adolescent years can affect our ability to trust others in the future.

We need to use both reason and emotion when we choose relationships. When we follow only our hearts we usually end up subconsciously choosing people who are similar to our parents, and we repeat the same patterns of betrayal. We don't realize we're choosing the same types of people over and over again, but we do so subconsciously in an attempt to recreate our childhood experiences but with the hope of a different outcome. Unfortunately we usually find ourselves with people who can't meet our needs and whose character and behaviour don't match our values. We trust them at first because they seem familiar to us, but their lack of ability to provide us with the dependability we need causes more relationship breakdowns and damage to our self-esteem.

How does trust relate to self-esteem?

Recent studies have shown a significant correlation between self-esteem and a person's ability to trust. Results of a further study on the relationship between trust and self-esteem showed that participants in the study had to trust themselves in their judgement of whom to trust and to accept themselves before they could ask another person to accept and trust them. What this means is that our ability and willingness to trust others is largely based on our ability to trust ourselves, and that self-trust comes from positive feelings of self-worth.

We can only really trust others when we feel good about ourselves. When our self-esteem increases, our levels of trust in our relationships also increase. A lack of trust in our relationships is a reflection of our fear of being hurt and betrayed again and a lack of ability to trust ourselves to cope with that possibility. When we learn to trust ourselves – and consequently become clearer about whom we should and shouldn't trust – our self-esteem increases.

When we have high self-esteem we feel more confident and have a greater sense of our own self-worth – we find it easier to trust others because if that trust is broken, we trust ourselves to have the strength to handle it. Even when we experience disappointment it doesn't affect our positive feelings about ourselves. When we have healthy self-esteem, we believe we're still worthy and loveable.

The mindful way – observing

A key element of mindfulness is observing, which is simply noticing what is happening right now. When we observe things, thoughts, feelings and situations, we see them as they truly are. In this way we can separate our past experiences – which created trust issues – from our fears about the future. We can leave the past in the past and focus on the present, seeing situations, experiences and people as they are. When we're observing mindfully we're letting go of our attachment to our trust issues and our autopilot reactions to the fear they generate. By focusing on observing the present we can make informed and conscious choices about whom to trust and what to trust.

In *Why Do I Do That?*, Joseph Burgo explains:

> Only by being vigilant – paying constant attention to yourself, observing your usual defences in action and then choosing not to engage in them whenever possible – will you be able to ease their hold upon you. Only by making a different choice, over and over, will you begin to develop new habits . . . you hone your skill through regular effort, just as you become a better musician with daily practice.

Our romantic relationships in particular draw out our subconscious fears and issues from the past. But when we make choices and act on those fears, such as choosing a relationship out of the fear of being alone, we're setting ourselves up for more hurt. Observing your behaviour, your choices and your patterns allows you to break out of the subconscious mode and make conscious choices based on what's best for you, instead of on fear. As Burgo suggests, we need to be observing and aware on a regular basis so we can make healthier choices again and again and free ourselves from the automatic response of unhealthy habits.

Mindfulness involves a detached observation of thoughts and emotions as they arise, which allows us to become aware of our own fears and worries and see them as separate and temporary objects rather than triggers to be acted upon. While we usually jump to conclusions, especially when it comes to matters of trust, mindful observation allows us to consider all the facts – like an impartial spectator – before we decide whom to trust and with whom to share our lives.

In a recent study on mindfulness and trust, Erika N. Carlson suggested that the non-judgemental observation and attention of mindfulness can help us see ourselves and know ourselves better. When we observe our thoughts, feelings and behaviour in a compassionate, non-judgemental way, we're able to let go of our fear-based reactions – such as denial, lying to ourselves for self-protection, feelings of inadequacy – and see ourselves as we truly are. With this clearer picture of who we are and what we're doing, we can make better choices.

> Tom had been practising mindful meditation for three weeks. He found it helped him to feel calmer and less reactive, especially when anxious or stressed. When he noticed his anxious feelings, he realized it was his fear about trust issues coming to the surface again. Whenever he could he took a moment simply to stop and breathe. He observed his anxiety, noticed his beating heart, became aware of how fearful he was. He knew he became anxious and angry whenever Susan was late home because he feared she was being unfaithful. But he could see now that that was a reaction to his past. His mother had been unfaithful to his father and it had torn their relationship apart. Grilling his wife when she came home was his way of trying to stop her from hurting him in the same way. But he was reacting to the past and not the present. In the present he could let those feelings go. Susan wasn't his mother, she was a separate person. And his feelings weren't about Susan. He took another deep breath and watched his anxiety and nervousness swirl around him like snow, until it stopped. He felt calmer, and decided he wouldn't question Susan; he'd work on trusting her.

Mountain meditation

When we're caught up in the drama of life we often try to think about the problem and come up with a rational solution. Using our thinking mind we analyse, make judgements and tell ourselves stories in an attempt to make sense of things. And yet our thinking mind is usually unfocused when we're in distress, making our thinking confused and creating more stress as we struggle to find a way out.

Our thinking mind is most helpful, says Carl Benedict, a counsellor, when we're operating from a calm and unemotional state. By switching from analysis to mindfulness we can bring ourselves to a calmer state, to becoming an observer. The observing self simply observes and accepts. It allows us to see what's going on and then respond appropriately, rather than reactively. Getting in touch with the observing self can only happen when you're calm enough to let go of the busy, noisy, restless thoughts swirling around in your mind. It's that chaotic state that leads us to feelings of low self-worth and the creation of emotional instability and stress.

One of the ways we can develop our observing skills is through mindfulness meditation practice. Jon Kabat-Zinn developed a mindfulness meditation called the Mountain Meditation. Its purpose is to help you become calm and grounded and access your observing self when you're faced with stressful and emotional circumstances. This meditation is designed to last about 20 minutes but can be shortened or extended based on your preference.

In this meditation, Kabat-Zinn suggests that just as a mountain is unaffected by the changing weather all around it, we all possess the same inner calm and strength that are unaffected by the thoughts and emotions and drama of our lives.

1 Sit down in a comfortable position on the floor or in a chair.
2 Breathe in and breathe out for a few moments, focusing your attention on your breath.
3 Imagine in vivid detail the most beautiful mountain you can think of. Picture the snow-capped peaks and rocks, the wildflowers in summer, the blue sky behind it.
4 Notice its stable, unmoving presence grounded in the earth.
5 After a few minutes of seeing this clear picture in your mind, imagine bringing the mountain inside yourself and becoming the mountain.
6 Imagine yourself sitting in stillness and in calm, like a mountain, simply observing and resting, unwavering as the various weather patterns, storms and seasons pass around you.
7 Just as a mountain endures constant changes and extremes, we also experience various thoughts, emotions and life challenges. Imagine viewing these experiences as external, fleeting and impersonal events, like temporary weather patterns.
8 Feel yourself being calm, strong and rooted in stillness amid the constant change of your internal and external experience.

By focusing on the observing self – that is, seeing yourself as an objective spectator instead of becoming immersed in the fear-based thoughts and feelings that lead you to make poor choices – you can feel calmer and see things more clearly. You can see whom to trust and whom not to trust. You can see yourself and the way you react and you can see other people, not as villains or angels but people with their own fears and vulnerabilities, just like you.

10

Materialism or non-attachment

For people with low self-esteem, objects become a way of demonstrating not only their sense of self, but their self-worth.

Tom and Susan were going out to a special event with Tom's work – a dinner with speeches and dancing afterwards. Susan was really looking forward to getting dressed up and going dancing but didn't know what to wear. She felt nothing she had was good enough. Most of the other couples were better off, and she didn't want to look frumpy – everyone would be looking at her and judging her. A week before, she and Tom got into a fight when she went out shopping for a new dress. She knew they couldn't really afford it but felt she'd done the right thing. As soon as she'd handed over her credit card she'd felt a rush of excitement, and felt so much better when she walked out with the designer-label shopping bag.

What is materialism?

Research shows that we all associate our possessions with ourselves. Having and possessing things supports our sense of who we are. In addition, possessions give us an opportunity to express our sense of identity to others. Whether it's a new pair of shoes or a new car, we use objects to tell the world – as well as ourselves – who we are and how we want to be perceived. We also believe that more or better possessions will lead to increased happiness.

Consumer researchers define materialism as 'the importance a consumer attaches to worldly possessions' and 'the importance a person places on possessions and their acquisition as a necessary or desirable form of conduct to reach desired end states, including happiness'. When we feel self-worth depends on a particular external standard, such as buying a certain electronic device, making a million dollars or getting accepted into a certain university, we feel good about ourselves when we meet those goals.

But the cost of associating our value as a person with external things and others' approval is high. Studies show that people who strongly value possessions and money have lower psychological well-being, including low life satisfaction and happiness, and more depression and anxiety, physical ailments and social problems.

In his book *The High Price of Materialism*, the psychologist Tim Kasser writes that materialistic values undermine our well-being because they perpetuate feelings of insecurity, weaken our connection to others and make us feel trapped.

We think there's so much more outside of us than inside, we pursue houses and cars and money because we think they'll make us feel safe and happy. But if we lose those things, we also feel we've lost a part of ourselves. When we become attached to things or the belief that we need to hold on to our wealth, fame, status or position, we can easily find ourselves feeling anxious, depressed, disappointed or worried that we'll lose them. What we thought would bring us happiness can quickly make us unhappy, and all too often we deal with that by trying to acquire even more.

Many people who are materialistic also become stingy – with both their possessions and their emotions. In an attempt to hold on to their fragile sense of self they can become selfish, hoarding love, emotions and things, taking without giving and offering only fragments of their heart, as if they were in short supply. 'The opposite of emotional generosity', writes Barbara De Angelis in *Are You the One for Me?*, 'is emotional stinginess.'

How does materialism relate to self-esteem?

For people with low self-esteem, objects become a way of demonstrating not only their sense of self, but their self-worth. Instead of deciding for themselves they're acceptable and loveable, they link their value to their possessions and allow others to judge their worth. In this way, people with low self-esteem can become obsessed with accumulating the right objects, the right job and the right praise and admiration from others, in order to feel loved and acceptable.

Researchers agree that accumulating material things is a way for people to try to deal with or compensate for their own insecurities and self-doubts about their safety, competence and self-worth. They rely upon certain products to boost their image of a tough guy, for example, or a beautiful woman, with the use of perfume, cars, clothing or designer labels. People with low self-esteem believe the value of certain objects enhances the value of the person associated with them.

But their positive feelings that arise with the accumulation of objects and external validation don't last long. As new challenges arise and positive feedback from others dwindles, their self-esteem can quickly fall again and they seek to regain others' approval with the acquisition of more possessions.

People with low self-esteem and high materialistic values can easily become 'caught in an endless cycle of acquiring material goods in the hope of compensating for feelings of insecurity and searching for happiness', say the researchers Lan Nguyen Chaplin and Deborah Roedder John in the *Journal of Consumer Research*. The happiness they actually find in the acquisition of material goods is short-lived and consequently leads them to try to resolve their stressful negative feelings about themselves by buying more things.

A study in the *Journal of Economic Psychology* showed that compulsive shoppers turn to shopping because they believe the purchases will boost their moods, rather as alcoholics turn to drink to feel better. They know it's not good for them but they like the initial 'high' and the sense of themselves as a person transformed.

Where does materialism come from?

People who are highly materialistic were often raised in non-nurturing environments that failed to provide for their needs for security and safety, writes Tim Kasser. Such environments tend to diminish people's self-esteem.

Kasser and his colleagues suggest that one way materialistic values develop is from experiences that induce feelings of insecurity. Many people become materialistic during the period between middle childhood and early adolescence. When children enter puberty, their self-esteem often takes a dip and they begin to pursue materialistic goals as a coping strategy. Studies suggest that children who experience chronically low self-esteem are more likely to express greater materialism over time.

Low self-esteem not only increases materialism, but being materialistic also lowers self-esteem. In a financial education programme designed to reduce materialism by lowering spending and promoting sharing and saving, students with high materialistic values who participated reported increased self-esteem over time, while those who didn't participate reported decreased self-esteem. In other words, the more they focused on spending and accumulating things, the lower their self-esteem became.

We also live in a very materialistic society filled with advertising that encourages us to spend more and buy things, assuring us we'll be happier and more fulfilled if we do. It's all too easy to compare ourselves with those around us and find ourselves lacking if we don't have the same quality of material possessions or status. This focus on materialism only serves to highlight our own sense of inadequacy, triggering negative thoughts and feelings about ourselves. According to Kasser:

> When people believe that their worth depends on external signifiers such as money and status, they are much more easily buffeted by the whims of fate than when they have a secure, stable, and deep sense of esteem that is not dependent on such accomplishments.

When we lose sight of the true value of ourselves without the need for external validation of our worth, we lose our individuality and our ability to cope and contribute to the world in a positive way.

The mindful way – non-attachment

Mindfulness provides a way of looking at things, people and feelings with a sense of non-attachment, which means we recognize they don't belong to us – they just are.

Non-attachment, or letting go, is the goal of Buddhism. Buddha taught that the cause of suffering is craving and attachment. By letting go we can alleviate the anxiety, stress, dissatisfaction and feelings of low self-worth that come with struggling for more.

With your own feelings, you recognize they're not a reflection of who you are and your worth, but temporary states. Thinking negative thoughts – such as 'I'm never going to reach my goals' or 'Why would anyone love me?' – quickly create negative feelings of depression and anxiety and lower your self-esteem.

But seeing emotions as transient and temporal and becoming unattached means you can allow yourself to experience them without trying to push them away, avoid them or cope with them by going shopping.

The negative emotions we feel often come from thinking about a past experience we want to hold on to or a future one we hope will bring us the happiness we seek. It can also be about trying to avoid or escape unpleasant thoughts or feelings. For many people, focusing on material things is a way of holding on to a positive view of themselves while avoiding unpleasant feelings. But trying to cling to experiences, things, people, feelings, beliefs, situations or habits only brings suffering.

'When we identify with our emotional states, thoughts, and perceptions of the world,' writes B. Raven Lee in *Attachment and Non-Attachment*, 'the result is rigidity, grasping onto a desired outcome, or pushing away what we fear.'

Non-attachment versus detachment

Non-attachment is not the same thing as detachment, says Joseph Goldstein, a meditation teacher. Being detached is distancing yourself from experience, pulling away and avoiding. But non-attachment means not holding on, not grasping. It's not suppressing your thoughts, feelings or desires but developing an awareness of your attachment to them and letting that attachment go. What this implies is that without attachment or grasping, we let go of struggling. When we stop struggling and just accept, we release ourselves from stress and despair and simply feel at peace.

The Zen teacher John Daido Loori explains that, according to Buddhism, non-attachment is the opposite of detachment or separation:

> You need two things in order to have attachment: the thing you're attaching to, and the person who's attaching. In non-attachment, on the other hand, there's unity. There's unity because there's nothing to attach to. You have unified with the whole universe.

Non-attachment means you can allow emotions to appear and then disappear without the need to try to change them. The harder you try to avoid them the harder they'll try to get your attention. Becoming non-attached means you stop defining yourself by the way you feel and stop trying to compensate by engaging in self-destructive behaviours, such as using material things to determine your worth. It's about being present and accepting your experiences, including your thoughts and feelings, rather than *identifying* yourself with them.

But it doesn't mean you don't care, you don't feel or you live disconnected from the world around you. Instead, you don't need to try and hold on to pleasant experiences or try to push away unpleasant experiences. In many ways you feel more, you experience more and your life becomes richer because you're more aware of feelings and experiences and don't try to either avoid them or attach yourself to them. Instead you cultivate a compassionate, non-judgemental view of your experiences, even in the face of challenges. In this way, says the Buddhist monk Ajahn Sucitto, non-attachment is presence, awareness, not absence.

Non-attachment and abundance versus addiction

Although it may seem contradictory, letting go of material things allows you to feel you have more. This is because you become aware of what you already have and appreciate it. When you're focused on gaining more things you lose awareness and instead focus on the craving, which makes you believe you *have* nothing and consequently you *are* nothing. You keep struggling to acquire more to fill that void inside you, but it's never enough. The space inside only grows emptier.

Attachment to material things is like an addiction. The high you get from the first hit, whether it's another new gadget or another drug, keeps you coming back for more. Materialism is an attempt to compensate with objects for the lack of love and acceptance you experienced growing up. But stuff will never be enough because it's not things that make you happy; it's not things that fill that emptiness inside you – it's love and acceptance.

What most people can't see is that it's not the lack of what you want that brings you unhappiness, but the yearning for it.

The next time Susan and Tom attended a special event, Susan decided to wear an outfit she had at home – she had several she'd hardly worn. She wanted to look nice but this time wanted to enjoy the party instead of worrying about what she looked like, what other people were wearing and how everyone might be judging her. She got ready, fixed her hair, put on her lipstick and then sat down for a few moments by herself and took a deep breath. She closed her eyes and took another deep breath, reminding herself it didn't matter what anyone thought about her – she was happy with who she was. She took another deep breath and exhaled, feeling the anxiety, the worry, the fear, fall away. She was ready to enjoy the party!

Non-attachment allows you to stop reaching for the bottle, the shopping, the stuff, and instead sit back and just breathe, knowing you already have what you're reaching for. In this way you can relax and stop struggling, stop yearning and craving and feeling there's something missing. You already have the love and acceptance that will fill that void. It doesn't come from things, being rich, famous or popular, or even from other people. It's not external, it's internal – it's there inside you. When difficulties arise you can go with the flow and feel confident in your ability to cope and adapt to change. You just have to see the beauty of who you are – see that you're that one precious thing you need, and love and accept yourself.

Mindful meditation practice

Through mindful meditation you learn to become aware that you're clinging to something and that letting go will bring you peace. You'll know and you'll feel that you're all right without holding on to anything. Once you let go you'll be free of the need for external things to fill up that empty space inside you. You'll see that you already have everything you need inside you. You're already all right, just as you are.

Research has shown that mindfulness meditation develops a part of the brain related to the development of secure attachment. With practice, meditation can therefore enable us to live in a state of caring compassion, for ourselves and others, in which we can embrace our internal and external experiences without judging them. When we feel secure with who we are, we can let go of our need to attach ourselves to material things.

The mindfulness meditation master B. H. Gunaratana suggests, in *Mindfulness in Plain English*, that once we begin to see ourselves as we are now, rather than the way we think we should be, changes will flow naturally. You don't have to struggle. Meditation is a way of helping you become aware of yourself as you are now, without illusion, judgement or resistance. It encourages you to accept yourself and let go of anger, jealousy and other negative emotions that drive you into self-destructive, automatic behaviour.

Mindful meditation cultivates your awareness of yourself and your experiences. Many of us move through our lives without any awareness of who we are or what we're doing, allowing our emotions and thoughts to control our lives. Meditation allows you to listen to your thoughts and feelings without attaching your sense of self-worth to them.

The mindful breathing in the meditation opposite allows you to become aware only of the present moment. Your breathing is happening now, and by concentrating on your breath you're not thinking of the past or even your past breath. You're not worrying about the future or the next breath. There's only the present moment. In this way you're retraining your mind to become aware of yourself in the present with calm, loving, compassionate acceptance and to let go of anything else.

This calm, peaceful state is temporary, says Gunaratana, and ends when the meditation ends. But these moments become stepping stones on the path that leads to a more peaceful, accepting and contented life.

1 To begin, find a comfortable and quiet place to sit and let yourself relax.
2 Breathe in and breathe out, but don't try to control your breathing. Instead, try to focus on the spontaneous movement of the breath, as if you're simply observing it. This isn't always easy, especially for a beginner, but try to let go and allow it to happen naturally.
3 Don't be discouraged if your mind wanders. If it does, recognize that you're worrying or distracted and then gently, without criticizing yourself, return your focus to your breathing.
4 Sometimes your own willpower may get in the way. Becoming aware of when it happens allows you to recognize your own need to be in control. With practice, your breathing will happen on its own and you'll feel no need to control it.
5 As you focus on your breathing and your concentration deepens, your breathing will slow down and you'll face fewer distractions from your mind. At this stage you'll begin to feel a sense of calm and freedom from the negative thoughts and emotions that had previously upset you. All the hurt, anger, greed, jealousy, anxiety and fear fade away.

11

Self-sabotage or devotion

In the beginner's mind there are many possibilities, but in the expert's there are few.

Shunryu Suzuki

Susan was beginning to think her mother was right about her, that she wasn't clever enough to succeed in work and should just focus on her home and family. She didn't know what to do, so thought it best to do what her mother said – she probably wouldn't make a very good businesswoman anyway.

That night Susan told Tom her plan to quit her job and focus on being a wife and mother. When he asked her why, she shrugged and told him it was for the best.

'I'm not smart enough to have a career,' she said.

'Who told you that?' asked Tom.

'No one. That's just what I think.'

'Are you sure?'

'Well,' said Susan, 'I suppose that's what my mother's always said. And I think she's right. I mean, I went to that meeting at work last week and no one even listened to me.'

'But you told me you felt so nervous about it you didn't even bother to prepare, and didn't express your opinions during it.'

'That's because I knew everyone would reject my ideas.'

Tom held Susan's hand. 'Do you think that's because you didn't prepare? Maybe if you had, you'd have had the confidence to speak out.'

Susan looked at him. 'Why on earth would I do that? Are you suggesting I did it on purpose?'

'No, I'm saying maybe you were expecting to fail, so you made sure you would. At least that way you'd be right.'

What is self-sabotage?

While low self-esteem often damages our relationships with our friends, family and colleagues, it tragically causes the most harm to ourselves. Low self-esteem often leads us to self-sabotage and to behave in ways that aren't in our own best interests. We push away the people who do care about us, develop relationships with people who don't, and let career opportunities slip through our fingers. In some cases we destroy our own happiness by abusing alcohol, overeating or overspending. In attempting to deal with a problem we tend to create more problems and place more obstacles in our way.

A study by Yu Niiya, Amara Brook and Jennifer Crocker illustrates how our self-esteem is tied to our willingness to sabotage ourselves. Participants were allowed to choose music before completing a written test. When the researchers reviewed the types of music chosen they found that those whose self-esteem was tied to their performance – rather than their own self-worth – actually chose music that was the most distracting. The study revealed that this act of sabotaging their success enabled them to blame the music if they performed poorly. In this way they could protect their self-esteem with the rationale that their failure was not their fault, but they were willing to jeopardize their ability to pass the test to do so. These findings show that when our self-esteem depends on our effort and performance, rather than ourselves as we are, we often choose to sacrifice our success in case our efforts aren't good enough.

Why do we sabotage ourselves?

People with low self-esteem often hold a deep-rooted belief that they don't deserve success or happiness or a loving relationship. When they experience positive emotions such as joy and love, says the psychotherapist Martha Baldwin, author of *Self-Sabotage*, they may feel so uncomfortable that they engage in self-sabotaging behaviour to bring about the results they believe they deserve.

Some people may have had so many experiences with failure and disappointment that they expect it to continue – they jeopardize promising situations to bring about the loss with which they're so familiar.

This deep-rooted belief in your own unworthiness usually starts in childhood. The messages – verbal and behavioural – you hear when you're growing up become part of your own inner dialogue. For example, if your parents told you you didn't do well in school because you were lazy, you'll tend to say the same thing to yourself whenever you're faced with a challenge that requires you to work hard. 'What's the point?' you say to yourself, 'I'll never succeed anyway.' Believing the negative comments and criticisms about you will lead you to act in ways that reinforce those beliefs, giving you evidence of your own failings and perpetuating the cycle of self-sabotage.

Likewise, says the psychologist and author Robert Firestone, children can adopt the self-defeating attitudes and behaviours their parents have about themselves. If parents feel insecure about their intelligence, for example, their children may grow up feeling they're not intelligent either, especially when parents continually make disparaging remarks about themselves, such as 'Why did I do that? I'm such an idiot!'

Self-sabotaging behaviour is usually subconscious, however, and most of us are completely unaware of the beliefs that hold us back, or of the ways we defeat ourselves. But we find ourselves continually drawn to self-sabotaging thoughts, beliefs and actions that make us unhappy because they allow us to feel the way we felt when we were growing up. And that sense of familiarity feels more comforting and safe than anything unfamiliar, even if the unfamiliar will bring us love, success and happiness.

How do we sabotage ourselves?

Although there are many ways we sabotage ourselves, according to the clinical psychologist Marilyn Sorensen they fall into two categories: underachievers and overachievers.

Underachievers

People in this category take whatever comes their way, without taking charge or direction of their own lives. Fearful of failure or rejection, they stay in low-paying, unfulfilling jobs and unhappy relationships with the belief that it's as good as it's going to get. They don't make the effort to improve their lives – such as taking classes, joining groups or getting help – because they fear they'll be criticized, judged, ridiculed or in some way found inadequate, confirming their worst fears. They continue to repeat their mistakes and negative patterns, unaware of their own self-defeating behaviour. Often dependent, they look to others for direction and defer to their opinions when they have to make choices. These are the people-pleasers who'll do anything to be liked, accepted and cared for, whether other people act in their best interests or not.

Overachievers

Some people with low self-esteem choose to put all their attention and energy into meeting their goals and can easily become workaholics. Their drive to succeed serves to give them a sense of accomplishment so they can feel good about themselves while also allowing them to avoid their painful emotional lives, where they feel hurt and inadequate. They justify their lack of a healthy personal life with the defence that they're too busy or too successful to manage the demands of a relationship, often ignoring or neglecting their loved ones.

Here are a few of the ways both under- and overachievers with low self-esteem try to avoid painful feelings and difficult situations in self-sabotaging ways:

- *Avoiding your feelings* Most people find facing painful feelings difficult. No one wants to admit to feeling scared, lonely or angry. But people with low self-esteem will regularly avoid dealing with or expressing their emotions, which provides temporary relief but tends to eliminate the possibility of true intimacy in relationships.
- *Self-medicating* Comfort eating, drinking too much and overspending are all ways you can try to make yourself feel better. But the effect is only temporary and you can quickly become addicted to the immediate high it brings – and ruin your health, finances and future in the process.
- *Procrastination* While it may seem harmless, procrastination is

the act of letting yourself down. You intend to do something and then avoid doing it, making excuses to justify your self-defeating behaviour. You stay in a job you hate, putting off looking for one you want. You tell yourself you didn't have the time or the money or the energy, but your actions are saying you're not worth the effort. And you believe it.

- *Keeping busy* You work hard, keep busy and find yourself struggling to get it all done, and feel proud of yourself for working so hard, even when you're not making any progress on what really matters to you. You can tell your friends and neighbours you worked late and baked a dozen brownies, which brings a pay-off of recognition and perhaps praise, but you know you're no closer to starting the novel or developing the business you really want.

- *Self-deprecation* A measure of modesty is a good thing, but when it becomes extreme you reject compliments, squander opportunities for advancement and fail to seize the moment when your voice might be heard. You do this by focusing your efforts on your failings, weaknesses and unimportant ideas, all of which serve to push you into the background of your own life.

- *Unhealthy relationships* Because people are attracted to what's familiar to them they often choose relationships that recreate the dynamics of their childhood, allowing them to maintain the negative self-image with which they've come to identify. You may rush too quickly into relationships or leave them abruptly when emotions develop. You may not believe happy relationships are possible so you instigate conflict when things are going well.

However self-sabotage manifests itself in your life, the result is that you end up getting in the way of your own happiness and obscuring the path to your own success. You can't change the past, but as an adult you can take control of your life and limit the ways the past controls you.

By identifying the negative beliefs that continually race through your mind and becoming aware of the self-sabotaging behaviours that keep you locked in a state of fear and frustration, you can let go of the past and move freely. In this way you can learn who you really are and what you really want. Instead of reacting to a patchwork of painful memories, damaging thoughts and unpleasant feelings, and fearing the future, you can live in the present. You can choose who you want to be and how you want to live your life.

In *The Self Under Siege*, Robert and Lisa Firestone and Joyce Catlett write that letting go of the grip of the past involves separating yourself from the destructive thoughts and beliefs you've internalized from your childhood. Once you've let go of the negative influence of the past that's weakened your self-esteem, you can begin to develop your own sense of self, including your own beliefs about who you are and what you want. You can develop your own values and begin to choose your own path through life, one day at a time, one moment at a time.

The mindful way – devoted

By encouraging you to focus on the moment, mindfulness gives you the tools to let go of the past and the negative thoughts that reinforce your self-destructive behaviour. Devotion is an important part of mindfulness because it allows you to live each day, each moment, in the enjoyment of your own being. When you're devoted to a mindful path, you're able to loosen the hold the past has on you and see your own true nature. Without devotion, you can too easily give up on yourself and the love that lives within you.

A devotional or reverential attitude allows you to see past your limited way of seeing the world and yourself and to expand your vision to incorporate possibility. When you continue to experience life the way you always have, with the same thoughts and beliefs and responses, you'll continue to experience the same outcome. Devotion allows you to break through those unconscious patterns and set a new course.

Mindfulness doesn't mean blind faith, however. It doesn't mean you adhere to a practice because you think you should. It's based on each individual's recognition of his or her ability to choose how to live. In doing so, you also need to recognize that others have their own choices to make and their own needs, and to accept all your differences.

'I think I want to keep working,' said Susan.

'Okay,' said Tom. 'Is that what you want?'

Susan realized she'd been living according to her mother's rules and ideas about who she was. Over time she'd become more concerned with getting people's attention and praise and affection than actually figuring out what she wanted to do with her life and what made her happy. It wasn't until she'd stopped trying so hard to please other people that she gave herself the chance to stop and just breathe. She'd decided to devote ten minutes a day to meditation and one hour a week to yoga. And now she could see the ways she was sabotaging her own success. She was smart enough to have a career, she just didn't believe she could do it. She'd actually created a life in which she was setting herself up for failure.

'I know what I want now,' she told Tom. 'I know no one else thinks I can do it, but I think I can.'

Tom smiled. 'I think you can too.'

Mindfulness practice

In the same way that we practise being the people others want us to be, repeating the old stories and the old thoughts from the past that reinforce our negative view of ourselves, over time a devotion to regular mindfulness practice can reinforce a positive sense of self.

When you participate in a formal daily practice of meditation, yoga, mindful walking or mindful breathing, and you live each moment mindfully, taking a moment to breathe consciously whenever your autopilot causes you to react, it's important to do so with a sense of devotion. With repeated practice, mindfulness can allow you to discover your own true nature and find the self-confidence to live the life you want to live.

Regular mindfulness practice not only increases your sense of calm and peacefulness, it also affects every aspect of your life, including your self-esteem and your ability to direct your own life. In *Zen Mind, Beginner's Mind*, the Zen master Shunryu Suzuki writes:

> While you are continuing this practice, week after week, year after year, your experience will become deeper and deeper, and your experience will cover everything you do in your everyday life . . . Do not think about anything. Just remain on your cushion without expecting anything. Then eventually you will resume

your own true nature. That is to say, your own true nature resumes itself.

Like regular exercise, setting up a regular mindfulness practice schedule, a certain time devoted to developing mindfulness, can allow you to feel the positive effects each time you participate as well as reap the rewards over the long term. It's not easy to train your mind to just sit and not think, especially after a lifetime of thinking and worrying and trying to distract yourself from unpleasant feelings and memories. But mindfulness is not about pushing thoughts away. It's facing them, acknowledging them and watching them drift away. It's seeing all the clutter in your mind as separate from yourself and losing your attachment to the pain and suffering they cause.

Every time you sit down and meditate you're giving yourself the gift of peace, an opportunity to weaken that attachment to negative beliefs and find a clear view of who you really are without the chaos of the past that's held you back for so long. It may feel strange and unusual just to sit and breathe, and it may be difficult at first to let go of the thoughts racing through your mind, but the more positively you feel about mindful practice, the more you'll get out of it. If you dread meditation, it won't help you, but if you look forward to it you'll be able to experience a greater sense of peace.

With repetition, the images of peace and tranquillity and love that begin to flow naturally into your mind during meditation will move from your conscious mind to your subconscious. The subconscious is where all the negative thoughts and feelings live because you've repeated them to yourself so many times. With practice the subconscious mind can instead be the home of positive feelings and thoughts and beliefs. Since it's your subconscious thoughts that drive your behaviour, with practice you'll behave in a way that doesn't sabotage your happiness and success, but seeks to fulfil you and bring you joy because it's driven not by fear but by the love and acceptance you've developed for yourself.

Devotional love

Devotion is central to the spiritual path, but we often find it difficult to be devoted because we feel we must put our rational minds in charge. We fear we might somehow lose ourselves by letting go.

Mindfulness can help you redirect your focus so you become attached to your true self rather than anything outside yourself. Through devotion to mindfulness you don't lose yourself, rather you lose the fear, anger, worry and anxiety that plague you instead of clinging to them. You allow yourself to cling to the essence of who you are, to your true self.

Perhaps our real fear is that we might find ourselves. For many people with low self-esteem, this is a frightening idea because they don't like themselves – they've spent their entire lives trying to avoid who they are. But the truth is that you don't even know your true self. You think you don't love who you are because you've been living as someone else's idea of who you are. Your sense of self is based on all kinds of negative ideas you've accepted as your identity. Once you let go of those thoughts and beliefs, your defences, rationalizations, emotional reactions and the self-sabotaging ways you perpetuate them, you're left with only your true self. And what you'll find is not fear, anger, shame, anxiety, self-doubt, control or hatred, but love.

For many people, it's easier to understand and accept the idea of romantic love or motherly love because it's the love for another. We often love someone or something because it gives us a sense of security or community, or to feel needed – this is only natural. On a deeper spiritual level you can let go of your ego, however, and love unconditionally, without any expectation. Without desire, fear or praise you can find inner peace.

And while it may feel strange and unfamiliar, you can also love yourself without the expectation that anyone or anything outside you will give you the love and peace you've always longed for. It's love without an object or an objective. It's the recognition of divine love within yourself.

Beginner's mind

A 'beginner's mind' is a way of experiencing life that's full of possibility and curiosity. When you have a beginner's mind you look at things as if you're seeing them for the first time, with openness and eagerness and freedom from expectation. By adopting a beginner's mind, even when you've been practising mindfulness for a long time, you can continue to see things in a new light rather than automatically responding to them with the same old patterns of behaviour.

Seeing the big picture and other perspectives and possibilities is essential to overcoming your self-sabotaging ways because you need to look beyond the limited view that kept you confined to limited possibilities. Again in the words of Shunryu Suzuki, 'In the beginner's mind there are many possibilities, but in the expert's there are few.'

As children we all have beginner's mind. We don't bring expectations or judgements or fear to our experiences, we simply see things as they are and marvel at their beauty. Even as adults we're beginners in some activities when we try something we've never done before. This is when we experience excitement and openness to learning and enjoy only the moment and the experience as they are.

Why do we lose our beginner's mind? When something becomes familiar to us, our minds try to help us by recalling similar experiences and memories and all the feelings – including fear, anxiety and doubt – we felt in previous experiences. Consequently we bring those feelings and memories and expectations, and block our experience of the present as it is. When we can live with a beginner's mind we can see the possibilities in everything. We're freeing ourselves from the limitations of the past, with its preconceived ideas and negative attitudes, and letting ourselves see things as they really are. In this way we can also see ourselves as we really are, free from the limiting views and influences of the past and the fears of the future.

Embracing a beginner's mind doesn't mean we let go of common sense or fail to plan for the future. We can do both – look at our experiences with a sense of openness and wonder *and* set goals. We can see ourselves as full of possibility and beauty and also choose the direction we want our lives to take. We simply need to take our lives one step at a time and enjoy the journey, making choices every day that will lead us to where we want to be, but focusing on the joy of living today. Letting go of what you think you should do, you can use your open beginner's mind to trust your intuition and choose what's right for you, one moment at a time. You no longer have to be perfect or faultless when you focus on the questions instead of the answers. In this way there's joy in *not* knowing, and simply being open to all the possibilities life holds.

Conclusion

When we use the tools of mindfulness and focus on the present moment, instead of the past or the future; when we develop an awareness of ourselves, our reactions, our thoughts and feelings and begin to see them objectively and non-judgementally; when we participate with devotion and non-attachment in the process of living our own lives according to our own needs and values, we're living mindfully. A mindful life can build our self-esteem one moment at a time whenever we remember to breathe and recognize that we have a choice – we can react out of fear or we can pause and choose love.

We must also remember to maintain balance in all things. We must strive for what is best for us but also be gentle with ourselves. We need to show compassion for others but also for ourselves. We must love and let ourselves be loved; accept and be accepted. And most of all, we must love and accept ourselves, as we are, whoever we are, because we all deserve to be loved.

References

Introduction

Breines, Juliana G. and Serena Chen, 'Self-Compassion Increases Self-Improvement Motivation', *Personality and Social Psychology Bulletin* 2012, vol. 38, no. 9, 1133–43.

Burgo, Joseph, *Why Do I Do That? Psychological Defense Mechanisms and the Hidden Ways they Shape our Lives*, Chapel Hill, NC: New Rise Press, 2012.

Carlson, Erika N., 'Overcoming the Barriers to Self-Knowledge: Mindfulness as a Path to Seeing Yourself as You Really Are', *Perspectives on Psychological Science* 2013, vol. 8, 173–86.

Condon, Paul, Gaëlle Desbordes, Willa B. Miller and David DeSteno, 'Meditation Increases Compassionate Responses to Suffering', *Psychological Science* 2013, vol. 24, no. 10, 2125–7.

Fennell, Melanie J. V., 'Depression, Low Self-Esteem and Mindfulness', *Behaviour Research and Therapy* 2004, vol. 42, no. 9, 1053–67.

Jacobs, T. L., P. R. Shaver, E. S. Epel, A. P. Zanesco, S. R. Aichele, D. A. Bridwell, E. L. Rosenberg, B. G. King, K. A. Maclean, B. K. Sahdra, M. E. Kemeny, E. Ferrer, B. A. Wallace and C. D. Saron, 'Self-reported Mindfulness and Cortisol During a Shamatha Meditation Retreat', *Health Psychology* 2013, vol. 32, no. 10, 1104–9.

Kabat-Zinn, Jon, *Wherever You Go, There You Are: Mindfulness Meditation for Everyday Life*, New York: Piatkus, 2004.

Lapsley, Daniel K. and Paul C. Stey, 'Id, Ego, and Superego' in V. S. Ramachandran (ed.), *Encyclopedia of Human Behavior*, 2nd edn, Elsevier, 2012.

McGonigal, Kelly, *The Willpower Instinct: How Self-Control Works, Why It Matters, and What You Can Do To Get More of It*, New York: Avery, 2011.

Sorensen, Marilyn, *Breaking the Chain of Low Self-Esteem*, Sherwood, OR: Wolf Publishing, 2006.

Tyrell, Mark, 'Top Ten Facts about Low Self-Esteem', *Uncommon Knowledge*. Retrieved 24 Sept. 2014, <www.self-confidence.co.uk/articles/top-ten-facts-about-low-self-esteem/>.

Wood, Joanne V., W. Q. Elaine Perunovic and John W. Lee, 'Positive Self-Statements: Power for Some, Peril for Others', *Journal of Psychological Science* 2009, vol. 20, no. 7, 860–6.

1 Self-loathing or self-compassion

Fennell, Melanie, 'Depression, Low Self-Esteem and Mindfulness', *Behaviour Research and Therapy* 2004, vol. 42, no. 9, 1053–67.

Germer, Christopher, 'Meditations', *Mindful Self-Compassion*. Retrieved 22 June 2014, <www.mindfulselfcompassion.org/meditations_downloads. php>.

Germer, Christopher, *The Mindful Path to Self-Compassion*, New York: The Guilford Press, 2009.

Gilbert, P. and S. Procter, 'Compassionate Mind Training for People with High Shame and Self-Criticism: Overview and Pilot Study of a Group Therapy Approach', *Clinical Psychology and Psychotherapy* 2006, vol. 13, no. 6, 353–79.

Neff, Kristin, 'Self-Compassion: An Alternative Conceptualization of a Healthy Attitude Toward Oneself', *Self and Identity* 2003, vol. 2, no. 2, 85–101.

Neff, Kristin, *Self-Compassion: The Proven Power of Being Kind to Yourself*, New York: William Morrow, 2011.

Orsillo, Susan M. and Lizabeth Roemer, *The Mindful Way Through Anxiety*, New York: The Guildford Press, 2011.

Parker-Pope, Tara, 'Go Easy on Yourself, A New Wave of Research Urges', *The New York Times*. Retrieved 20 June 2014 <http://well.blogs.nytimes. com/2011/02/28/go-easy-on-yourself-a-new-wave-of-research-urges/>.

Rubin, Theodore I., *Compassion and Self-Hate*, Upper Saddle River, NJ: Prentice Hall, 1998.

Senay, I., D. Albarracín and K. Noguchi, 'Motivating Goal-Directed Behavior Through Introspective Self-Talk: The Role of the Interrogative Form of Simple Future Tense', *Psychological Science* 2010, vol. 21, no. 4, 499–504.

Shapiro, Shauna, 'Does Mindfulness Make You More Compassionate?', *Greater Good: The Science of Meaningful Life*. Retrieved 16 July 2014, <http://greatergood.berkeley.edu/article/item/does_mindfulness_make_ you_compassionate>.

White, Mark D., 'Do the Self-Loathing See the Same "Self" that Others Do?' *Psychology Today*. Retrieved 20 June 2014, <www.psychologytoday.com/ blog/maybe-its-just-me/201306/do-the-self-loathing-see-the-same-self-others-do>.

White, Mark D., 'Can Self-Compassion Help the Self-Loathing Person?', *Psychology Today*. Retrieved 20 June 2014, <www.psychologytoday.com/ blog/maybe-its-just-me/201103/can-self-compassion-help-the-self-loathing-person>.

2 Unhealthy relationships or living in the moment

Brach, Tara, 'Decide on Love: We Can Decide on Love, if We Are Able to Stay Present', *Psychology Today*. Retrieved 31 May 2014, <www.psychologytoday.com/blog/finding-true-refuge/201403/decide-love>.

Burgo, Joseph, *Why Do I Do That? Psychological Defense Mechanisms and the Hidden Ways They Shape our Lives*, Chapel Hill, NC: New Rise Press, 2012.

Chödrön, Pema, *When Things Fall Apart: Heart Advice for Difficult Times*, Rockport, MA: Element, 2005.

Dixit, Jay, 'The Art of Now: Six Steps to Living in the Moment', *Psychology Today*. Retrieved 16 May 2014, <www.psychologytoday.com/articles/200810/the-art-now-six-steps-living-in-the-moment>.

Gunaratana, B. H., *Mindfulness in Plain English*, Boston, MA: Wisdom Publications, 1996.

Jones, Ian Ellis, 'How to Live Moment to Moment', *Mindful*. Retrieved 12 May 2014, <www.mindful.org/mindfulness-practice/mindfulness-and-awareness/moment-to-moment>.

Kabat-Zinn, Jon, *Full Catastrophe Living: Using the Wisdom of your Mind to Face Stress, Pain and Illness*, New York: Dell Publishing, 1990.

Kabat-Zinn, Jon, 'Mindfulness of this Moment', *Living Life Fully*. Retrieved 10 May 2014, <www.livinglifefully.com/flo/flobemindfulnessofthismoment.htm>.

Lazar, S. W., C. E. Kerr, R. H. Wasserman, J. R. Gray, D. N. Greve, M. T. Treadway, M. McGarvey, B. T. Quinn, J. A. Dusek, H. Benson, S. L. Rauch, C. I. Moore and B. Fischl, 'Meditation Experience Is Associated with Increased Cortical Thickness', *NeuroReport* 2005, vol. 28, no. 16, 1893–7.

Lucas, Marsha, *Rewire Your Brain for Love: Creating Vibrant Relationships Using the Science of Mindfulness*, Carlsbad, CA: Hay House, 2013.

Luders, Eileen, Florian Kurth, Emeran A. Mayer, Arthur W. Toga, Katherine L. Narr and Christian Gaser, 'The Unique Brain Anatomy of Meditation Practitioners: Alterations in Cortical Gyrification', *Frontiers in Human Neuroscience*, 29 February 2012.

Meyers, Seth, *Dr. Seth's Love Prescription: Overcome Relationship Repetition Syndrome and Find the Love You Deserve*, Avon, MA: Adams Media, 2011.

Murray, Sandra L., John G. Holmes and Dale W. Griffin, 'Self-esteem and the Quest for Felt Security: How Perceived Regard Regulates Attachment Processes', *Journal of Personality and Social Psychology* 2000, vol. 78, no. 3, 478–98.

Murray, Sandra L., John G. Holmes, Dale W. Griffin, Gina Bellavia and Paul Rose, 'The Mismeasure of Love: How Self-Doubt Contaminates Relationship Beliefs', *Personal and Social Psychology Bulletin* 2001, vol. 27, no. 4, 423–36.

Nhat Hanh, Thich, *Stepping into Freedom: Rules of Monastic Practice for Novices*, Berkeley, CA: Parallax Press, 1997.

Nhat Hanh, Thich, 'Thich Nhat Hanh on the Practice of Mindfulness', *Shambhala Sun*, 1 March 2010. Retrieved 28 Oct. 2014, <www.lionsroar.com/mindful-living-thich-nhat-hanh-on-the-practice-of-mindfulness-march-2010/>.

Norwood, Robin, *Women Who Love Too Much*, Los Angeles, CA: Jeremy P. Tarcher, 1985.

Schueller, S., 'Preferences for Positive Psychology Exercises', *Journal of Positive Psychology* 2010, 5, 192–203.

Siegel, Daniel, *The Mindful Brain: Reflection and Attunement in the Cultivation of Well-Being*, New York: W. W. Norton, 2007.
Sorensen, Marilyn, *Breaking the Chain of Low Self-Esteem*, Sherwood, OR: Wolf Publishing, 2006.

3 Defensiveness or awareness

Barnes, Sean, Kirk Warren Brown, Elizabeth Krusemark, W. Keith Campbell and Ronald D. Rogge, 'The Role of Mindfulness in Romantic Relationship Satisfaction and Responses to Relationship Stress', *Journal of Marital and Family Therapy* 2007, vol. 33, no. 4, 482–500.
Burgo, Joseph, *Why Do I Do That? Psychological Defense Mechanisms and the Hidden Ways They Shape our Lives*, Chapel Hill, NC: New Rise Press, 2012.
Cobb, Nathan, *How to Overcome Defensiveness*, Retrieved 16 May 2014, <www.nathancobb.com/support-files/overcoming-defensiveness.pdf>.
Dingfelder, Sadie F., 'Tibetan Buddhism and Research Psychology: A Match Made in Nirvana? Collaborations Between Monks and Psychologists Yield New Directions in Psychological Research', *Monitor on Psychology* 2003, vol. 34, no. 11, 46.
Flowers, Steve, *The Mindful Path through Shyness: How Mindfulness and Compassion Can Help Free You from Social Anxiety, Fear and Avoidance*, Oakland, CA: New Harbinger, 2009.
Freud, Anna, *The Ego and the Mechanisms of Defence*, trans. Baines, Cecil, London: Hogarth Press and Institute of Psycho-Analysis, 1937.
Freud, Sigmund, 'The neuro-psychoses of defence' (1894), *The Standard Edition of the Complete Psychological Works of Sigmund Freud*, London: Hogarth Press, 1968.
Goldstein, Elisha, '7 Ways to Mindfully Boost Self-Esteem', *PsychCentral*. Retrieved 17 May 2014, <http://blogs.psychcentral.com/mindfulness/2009/05/7-ways-to-mindfully-boost-self-esteem/>.
Gottman, John, *Why Marriages Succeed or Fail: And How You Can Make Yours Last*, New York: Simon & Schuster, 1995.
Gunaratana, B. H., *Mindfulness in Plain English*, Boston, MA: Wisdom Publications, 1996.
Johnson, Sue, *Hold Me Tight: Seven Conversations for A Lifetime of Love*, New York: Little, Brown and Company, 2008.
Kabat-Zinn, Jon, *Full Catastrophe Living: Using the Wisdom of your Mind to Face Stress, Pain and Illness*, New York: Dell Publishing, 1990.
Nhat Hanh, Thich, *Peace is Every Step: The Path of Mindfulness in Everyday Life*, New York: Bantam, 1992.
Senay, I., D. Albarracín and K. Noguchi, 'Motivating Goal-Directed Behavior Through Introspective Self-Talk: The Role of the Interrogative Form of Simple Future Tense', *Psychological Science* 2010, vol. 21, no. 4, 499–504.

4 Control or acceptance

Alexander, Ronald, *Wise Mind, Open Mind: Finding Purpose and Meaning in Times of Crisis, Loss, and Change*, Oakland, CA: New Harbinger, 2009.

Burgo, Joseph, *Why Do I Do That? Psychological Defense Mechanisms and the Hidden Ways They Shape our Lives*, Chapel Hill, NC: New Rise Press, 2012.

Decker, David, J., 'What do You Mean I'm Being Controlling? Gaining a Better Understanding of What Control is and How it Affects You and Others Around You', *Anger Resources*. Retrieved 7 June 2014, <www.angeresources.com/controlarticle.html>.

Fitzgibbons, Richard, 'The Controlling and Mistrustful Spouse', *MaritalHealing.com*. Retrieved 6 June 2014, <www.maritalhealing.com/conflicts/controllingspouse.php>.

Gilbertson, Tina, 'Self-esteem and the Myth of not Needing Others', *GoodTherapy*. Retrieved 7 June 2014, <www.goodtherapy.org/blog/self-esteem-myth-of-not-needing-others/>.

Harris, A. H., F. M. Luskin, S. V. Benisovich, S. Standard, J. Bruning, S. Evans and C. Thoresen, 'Effects of a Group Forgiveness Intervention on Forgiveness, Perceived Stress and Trait Anger: A Intervention on Forgiveness, Perceived Stress and Trait Anger: A Randomized Trial', *Journal of Clinical Psychology* 2006, vol. 62, no. 6, 715–33.

Kaplan, Jeffrey, 'Control Issues', *Good Therapy*. Retrieved 18 May 2014, <www.goodtherapy.org/therapy-for-control-issues.html#>.

Kozak, Arnie, 'Acceptance is Mindfulness; Mindfulness is Acceptance', *Beliefnet*. Retrieved 12 June 2014, <www.beliefnet.com/columnists/mindfulnessmatters/2011/11/acceptance-is-mindfulness-mindfulness-is-acceptance.html>.

Parrott, Les, *The Control Freak: Coping with Those Around You, Taming the One Within*, Carol Stream, IL: Tyndale House, 2001.

Samsel, Michael, 'Subtly Controlling Behaviour', *Abuse and Relationships*. Retrieved 6 June 2014, <www.abuseandrelationships.org/Content/Behaviors/subtle_control.html>.

5 Perfectionism or non-judgement

Adderholdt-Elliott, Miriam, *Perfectionism: What's Bad About Being Too Good?*, Minneapolis, MN: Free Spirit Publishing, 1987.

Benson, Etienne, 'The Many Faces of Perfectionism', *Monitor on Psychology* 2003, vol. 34, no. 10, 18.

Burgo, Joseph, *Why Do I Do That? Psychological Defense Mechanisms and the Hidden Ways They Shape our Lives*, Chapel Hill, NC: New Rise Press, 2012.

Cobb, Nathan, *How to Overcome Defensiveness*. Retrieved 16 May 2014, <www.nathancobb.com/support-files/overcoming-defensiveness.pdf>.

Dogen Zenji, quoted in Elisha Goldstein, *Mindfulness Meditations for the*

Anxious Traveler: Quick Exercises to Calm Your Mind, New York: Simon & Schuster, 2012.

Frost, Randy O., Patricia Marten, Cathleen Lahart and Robin Rosenblate, 'The Dimensions of Perfectionism', *Cognitive Therapy and Research* 1990, vol. 14, no. 5, 449–68.

Frost, Randy O., Richard G. Heimberg, Craig S. Holt, Jill I. Mattia and Amy L. Neubauer, 'A Comparison of Two Measures of Perfectionism', *Personality and Individual Differences* 1993, vol. 14, no. 1, 119–26.

Gladding, Rebecca, 'Mindfulness is Judgmental', *Psychology Today*. Retrieved 12 June 2014, <www.psychologytoday.com/blog/use-your-mind-change-your-brain/201106/mindfulness-is-judgmental>.

Goldstein, Elisha, 'Seeing the Person: 4 Steps to End Judgmental Thoughts', *Huffington Post*. Retrieved 19 June 2014, <www.huffingtonpost.com/elisha-goldstein-phd/4-steps-to-better-relatio_b_779168.html>.

Gunaratana, B. H., *Mindfulness in Plain English*, Boston, MA: Wisdom Publications, 1996.

Hewitt, Paul L. and Gordon L. Flett, 'Perfectionism in the Self and Social Contexts: Conceptualization, Assessment and Association with Psychopathology', *Journal of Personality and Social Psychology* 1991, 60, 456–70.

Hewitt, Paul L., Gordon L. Flett, Simon B. Sherry, Marie Habke, Melanie Parkin, Raymond W. Lam, Bruce McMurtry, Evelyn Ediger, Paul Fairlie and Murray B. Stein, 'The Interpersonal Expression of Perfection: Perfectionistic Self-Presentation and Psychological Distress', *Journal of Personality and Social Psychology* 2003, vol. 84, no. 6, 1303–25.

Matta, Christy, 'Exercises for Non-judgmental Thinking', *PsychCentral*. Retrieved 12 June 2014, <http://blogs.psychcentral.com/dbt/2010/06/exercises-for-non-judgmental-thinking/>.

Zwolinski, Richard and C. R. Zwolinski, 'Top 5 Dangers of Being a Perfectionist', *PsychCentral*. Retrieved 12 June 2014, <http://blogs.psychcentral.com/therapy-soup/2014/06/top-5-dangers-of-being-a-perfectionist/>.

6 Criticism or compassion

Dalai Lama, *The Power of Compassion*, New York: HarperCollins, 1995.

Dalai Lama, *An Open Heart: Practising Compassion in Everyday Life*, ed. N. Vreeland, London: Hodder & Stoughton, 2001.

DeSteno, David, 'Compassion Made Easy', *The New York Times*. Retrieved 14 July 2014, <www.nytimes.com/2012/07/15/opinion/sunday/the-science-of-compassion.html?_r=1&>.

Gannett, Andrea Kay, 'At Work: To Succeed, Learn to Take Criticism', *USA Today*. Retrieved 8 July 2014, <www.usatoday.com/story/money/columnist/kay/2013/02/15/at-work-criticism-sensitivity/1921903/>.

Gilbert, Paul and Sue Procter, 'Compassionate Mind Training for People with High Shame and Self-Criticism: Overview and Pilot Study of a Group Therapy Approach', *Clinical Psychology and Psychotherapy* 2006, vol. 13, no. 6, 353–79.

Gilbertson, Tina, 'Self-Esteem and the Myth of Not Needing Others', *GoodTherapy.* Retrieved 7 June 2014, <www.goodtherapy.org/blog/self-esteem-myth-of-not-needing-others/>.

Gottman, John, *The Seven Principles for Making Marriage Work*, New York: Three Rivers Press, 1999.

Henry, William P., Thomas E. Schacht and Hans H. Strupp, 'Patient and Therapist Introject, Interpersonal Process, and Differential Psychotherapy Outcome', *Journal of Consulting and Clinical Psychology* 1990, vol. 58, no. 6, 768–74.

Holmes, Lindsay, '8 Ways to Tell if You're a *Truly* Compassionate Person', *Huffington Post.* Retrieved 19 June 2014, <http://www.huffingtonpost.com/2014/06/27/habits-of-compassionate-people_n_5522941.html>.

Keltner, Dacher, Jason Marsh and Jeremy Adam Smith, *The Compassionate Instinct: The Science of Human Goodness*, New York: W. W. Norton, 2010.

Nhat Hanh, Thich, *Interbeing: Fourteen Guidelines for Engaged Buddhism*, Berkeley, CA: Parallax Press, 1987.

Prior, Elly, 'Dealing with Criticism', *ProfessionalCounselling.* Retrieved 7 July 2014, <www.professional-counselling.com/dealing_with_criticism_rejection.html>.

Raven-Lee, B., 'Attachment and Non-Attachment: A Conversation between Buddhism and Psychology', *Connections and Reflections: The GAINS Quarterly* 2006, vol. 1, no. 4, 1–45.

Rosenthal, Neil, 'Why Do Critical People Get Angry When They Are Criticised?' *HeartRelationships.* Retrieved 7 July 7 2014, <http://heartrelationships.com/why-do-critical-people-get-angry-when-they-are-criticised/>.

Wallmark, Erik, Kousha Safarzadeh, Daiva Daukantaitė and Rachel E. Maddux, 'Promoting Altruism Through Meditation: An 8-Week Randomized Controlled Pilot Study', *Mindfulness* 2013, vol. 4, no. 3, 223–34.

Weng, Helen Y., Andrew S. Fox, Alexander J. Shackman, Diane E. Stodola, Jessica Z. K. Caldwell, Matthew C. Olson, Gregory M. Rogers and Richard J. Davidson, 'Compassion Training Alters Altruism and Neural Responses to Suffering', *Psychological Science* 21 May 2013, doi: 10.1177/0956797612469537.

7 People-pleasing or connected

Braiker, Harriet B., *The Disease to Please: Curing the People-Pleasing Syndrome*, New York: McGraw-Hill, 2011.

Earley, Jay, 'The People-Pleasing Pattern', *PersonalGrowthPrograms.*

Retrieved 4 Aug. 2014, <http://personal-growth-programs.com/people-pleasing/>.

Fine, Micki, *The Need to Please: Mindfulness Skills to Gain Freedom from People Pleasing and Approval Seeking*, Oakland, CA: New Harbinger, 2013.

Seltzer, Leon F., 'From Parent-Pleasing to People-Pleasing: How Craving Others' Approval Can Sabotage Healthy Self-Development', *Psychology Today*. Retrieved 8 July 2014, <www.psychologytoday.com/blog/evolution-the-self/200807/parent-pleasing-people-pleasing-part-1-3>.

Seppala, Emma, 'Connect to Thrive: Social Connection Improves Health, Well-Being and Longevity', *Psychology Today*. Retrieved 4 Aug. 2014, <www.psychologytoday.com/blog/feeling-it/201208/connect-thrive>.

Sorensen, Marilyn, *Breaking the Chain of Low Self-Esteem*, Sherwood, OR: Wolf Publishing, 2006.

Thich Nhat Hanh, *The Art of Power*, New York: HarperCollins, 2008.

8 Lack of assertiveness or participation

Amaro, Ajahn, 'Inner Listening', Amaravati Buddhist Monastery, Hemel Hempstead, Hertfordshire, 2012. Retrieved 26 Aug. 2014, <www.amara vati.org/downloads/pdf/Inner_Listening_-_Ajahn_Amaro.pdf>.

'Assertiveness', *Better Health Channel*. Retrieved 28 Aug. 2014, <www.betterhealth.vic.gov.au/bhcv2/bhcarticles.nsf/pages/Assertiveness>.

Boyce, Barry, 'The Healing Power of Mindfulness' (interview with Jon Kabat-Zinn, *Mindful.org*). Retrieved 20 Aug. 2014, <www.mindful.org/in-body-and-mind/health-and-healing/the-healing-power-of-mindfulness>.

Centre for Clinical Interventions, 'Assert Yourself!'. Retrieved 15 Aug. 2014, <www.cci.health.wa.gov.au/resources/infopax.cfm?Info_ID=51>.

Earley, Jay, 'The People-Pleasing Pattern', *Personal Growth Programs*. Retrieved 4 August 2014, <http://personal-growth-programs.com/people-pleasing/>.

Linehan, Marsha M., *DBT® Skills Training Manual*, 2nd edn, New York: The Guilford Press, 2014.

Pandita, Sayadaw U, 'How to Practice Vipassana Insight Meditation'. *Shambhala Sun*. Retrieved 29 Aug. 2014, <www.shambhalasun.com/index.php?option=content&task=view&id=1465>.

Seltzer, Leon F., 'Afraid to Rage: The Origins of Passive-Aggressive Behavior', *Psychology Today*. Retrieved 15 Aug. 2014, <www.psychologytoday.com/blog/evolution-the-self/200806/afraid-rage-the-origins-passive-aggressive-behavior>.

Smalley, Susan, 'Mindfulness Meditation – Achieving "Unentangled Participation"', *Huffington Post*. Retrieved 26 Aug. 2014, <www.huffing tonpost.com/susan-smalley/mindfulness-meditation_b_521585.html>.

Sorensen, Marilyn, *Breaking the Chain of Low Self-Esteem*, Sherwood, OR: Wolf Publishing, 2006.

9 Distorted sense of trust or observing

Benedict, Carl, 'Mindfulness: Paying Attention to Your Life', *Serenity Online Therapy*. Retrieved on 21 June 2014, <http://serenityonlinetherapy.com/mindfulness.htm>.

Burgo, Joseph, *Why Do I Do That? Psychological Defense Mechanisms and the Hidden Ways They Shape our Lives*, Chapel Hill, NC: New Rise Press, 2012.

Carlson, Erika N., 'Overcoming The Barriers to Self-Knowledge: Mindfulness as a Path to Seeing Yourself as You Really Are', *Perspectives on Psychological Science* 2013, vol. 8, no. 2, 173–86.

Cloud, Henry, *Integrity*, New York: HarperCollins, 2006.

Cloud, Henry and John Townsend, *Safe People*, Grand Rapids, MI: Zondervan, 1995.

Kabat-Zinn, Jon, *Wherever You Go, There You Are: Mindfulness Meditation for Everyday Life*, New York: Piatkus, 2004.

McDonagh, P., 'Shared Benefits: Group Therapy Delivers Open Honest Talk with People You Trust', *Chatelaine* 1997, vol. 70, 136.

Murray, S. L., R. T. Pinkus, J. G. Holmes, B. Harris, S. Gomillion, M. Aloni and S. Leder, 'Signaling When (And When Not) to Be Cautious and Self-Protective: Impulsive and Reflective Trust in Close Relationships', *Journal of Personality and Social Psychology* 2011, vol. 101, no. 3, 485–502.

Sorensen, Marilyn, *Breaking the Chain of Low Self-Esteem*, Sherwood, OR: Wolf Publishing, 2006.

Weining, Ashlee N. and Elizabeth L. Smith, 'Self-Esteem and Trust: Correlation Between Self-Esteem and Willingness to Trust in Undergraduate Students', *Student Pulse* 2012, vol. 4, no. 8.

Williams, Keith L. and Renee V. Galliher, 'Predicting Depression and Self-Esteem from Social Connectedness, Support, and Competence', *Journal of Social and Clinical Psychology* 2006, vol. 25, no. 8, 855–74.

Zak, A. M., J. A. Gold, R. M. Ryckman and E. Lenney, 'Assessments of Trust in Intimate Relationships and the Self-Perception Process', *The Journal of Social Psychology* 1998, vol. 138, no. 2, 217–28.

10 Materialism or non-attachment

Belk, Russell W., 'Possessions and the Extended Self', *Journal of Consumer Research* 1988, vol. 15, no. 2, 139–68.

Burkeman, Oliver, 'This Column Will Change Your Life' (Interview with Joseph Goldstein) *The Guardian*, Saturday, 4 July 2009. Retrieved 7 Aug. 2014, <www.theguardian.com/lifeandstyle/2009/jul/04/self-help-burkeman>.

Chaplin, L. N. and D. R. John, 'Growing up in a Material World: Age Differences in Materialism in Children and Adolescents', *Journal of Consumer Research* 2007, vol. 34, no. 4, 480–93.

De Angelis, Barbara, *Are You The One For Me? Knowing Who's Right and Avoiding Who's Wrong*, New York: Dell, 1992.

Donnelly, Grant, Masha Ksendzova and Ryan T. Howell, 'Sadness, Identity, and Plastic in Over-Shopping: The Interplay of Materialism, Poor Credit Management, and Emotional Buying Motives in Predicting Compulsive Buying', *Journal of Economic Psychology* 2013, vol. 39, 113–25.

Goldstein, Joseph and Jack Kornfield, *Seeking the Heart of Wisdom: The Path of Insight Meditation*, Boston, MA: Shambhala, 1987.

Gunaratana, B. H., *Mindfulness in Plain English*, Boston, MA: Wisdom Publications, 1996.

Kasser, Tim, *The High Price of Materialism*, Cambridge, MA: MIT Press, 2003.

Kasser, T., K. L Rosenblum, A. J. Sameroff et al., 'Changes in Materialism, Changes in Psychological Well-Being: Evidence from Three Longitudinal Studies and an Intervention Experiment', *Motivation and Emotion* 2014, vol. 38, no. 1, 22.

Lee, B. Raven, 'Attachment and Non-Attachment: A Conversation between Buddhism and Psychology' *Connections & Reflections: The GAINS Quarterly* 2006, vol. 1, no. 4, 1–45.

Loori, John Daido, 'The Whole Earth Is Medicine', *Mountain Record*, Spring 2004, vol. 22, no. 3.

Sucitto, Achaan, 'Non-Attachment Is Presence, Not Absence', Dharma Talk presented on *Dharma Seed*. Retrieved 11 Aug. 2014, <http://dharmaseed.org/teacher/9/talk/386/>.

11 Self-sabotage or devotion

Baldwin, Martha, *Self-Sabotage: How to Stop It and Soar to Success*, New York: Grand Central Publishing, 1990.

Baldwin Beveridge, Martha, *Meeting and Mastering your Internal Saboteur*, Options Now, 1994.

Campbell, Polly, 'End the Self-Sabotage to Make Good on Your Dreams', *Psychology Today*. Retrieved 17 Sept. 2014, <www.psychologytoday.com/blog/imperfect-spirituality/201304/end-the-self-sabotage-make-good-your-dreams>.

Firestone, Robert, Lisa Firestone and Joyce Catlett, *The Self Under Siege*, New York: Routledge, 2012.

Jaksch, Mary, 'How to Live Life to the Max with Beginner's Mind', *ZenHabits*. Retrieved 24 Sept. 2014, <http://zenhabits.net/how-to-live-life-to-the-max-with-beginners-mind/>.

Niiya, Y., A. T. Brook and J. Crocker, 'Contingent Self-Worth And Self-Handicapping: Do Contingent Incremental Theorists Protect Self-Esteem?', *Self and Identity* 2010, vol. 9, no. 3, 276–97.

Nithyananda, Paramahamsa, 'What Is a Beginner's Mind?', *Nithyananda.org*.

Retrieved 22 Sept. 2014, <www.nithyananda.org/article/what-beginner-mind#gsc.tab=0>.

Selby, Edward A., Timothy Pychyl, Hara Estroff Marano and Adi Jaffe, 'Self-Sabotage: The Enemy Within', *Psychology Today*. Retrieved 6 Sept. 2014, <www.psychologytoday.com/collections/201207/are-you-sabotaging-yourself/self-sabotage-the-enemy-within>.

Sorensen, Marilyn, *Breaking the Chain of Low Self-Esteem*, Sherwood, OR: Wolf Publishing, 2006.

Suzuki, Shunryu, *Zen Mind, Beginner's Mind: Informal Talks on Zen Meditation and Practice*, Boston, MA: Shambhala Publications, 2011.

Thera, Nyanaponika, 'Devotion in Buddhism', *Access to Insight (Legacy Edition)*. Retrieved 17 Sept. 2014, <www.accesstoinsight.org/lib/authors/nyanaponika/devotion.html>.

Index